COPING WITH

MARY-CLAIRE MASON is a [...] special interest in health. She is [...] Journalists' Association and The [...] She has written for the nation[...] women's magazines such as *Bella*, *Woman's Realm*, and *Essentials*. She lives in London with her husband, two cats and two Dalmatian dogs.

Overcoming Common Problems Series

For a full list of titles please contact
Sheldon Press, Marylebone Road, London NW1 4DU

The Assertiveness Workbook
A plan for busy women
JOANNA GUTMANN

Beating the Comfort Trap
DR WINDY DRYDEN AND JACK
GORDON

Birth Over Thirty Five
SHEILA KITZINGER

Body Language
How to read others' thoughts by their
gestures
ALLAN PEASE

Body Language in Relationships
DAVID COHEN

Calm Down
How to cope with frustration and anger
DR PAUL HAUCK

Cancer – A Family Affair
NEVILLE SHONE

The Candida Diet Book
KAREN BRODY

Caring for Your Elderly Parent
JULIA BURTON-JONES

Comfort for Depression
JANET HORWOOD

Coping Successfully with Hayfever
DR ROBERT YOUNGSON

Coping Successfully with Migraine
SUE DYSON

Coping Successfully with Pain
NEVILLE SHONE

Coping Successfully with PMS
KAREN EVENNETT

Coping Successfully with Panic Attacks
SHIRLEY TRICKETT

**Coping Successfully with Prostate
Problems**
ROSY REYNOLDS

**Coping Successfully with Your Irritable
Bladder**
JENNIFER HUNT

**Coping Successfully with Your Irritable
Bowel**
ROSEMARY NICOL

**Coping Successfully with Joint
Replacement**
DR TOM SMITH

Coping with Anxiety and Depression
SHIRLEY TRICKETT

Coping with Blushing
DR ROBERT EDELMANN

Coping with Breast Cancer
DR EADIE HEYDERMAN

Coping with Bronchitis and Emphysema
DR TOM SMITH

Coping with Candida
SHIRLEY TRICKETT

Coping with Chronic Fatigue
TRUDIE CHALDER

Coping with Cystitis
CAROLINE CLAYTON

Coping with Depression and Elation
DR PATRICK McKEON

Coping with Eczema
DR ROBERT YOUNGSON

Coping with Endometriosis
JO MEARS

Coping with Psoriasis
PROFESSOR RONALD MARKS

Coping with Schizophrenia
DR STEVEN JONES AND DR FRANK
TALLIS

Coping with Stomach Ulcers
DR TOM SMITH

Coping with Thyroid Problems
DR JOAN GOMEZ

Coping with Thrush
CAROLINE CLAYTON

Coping with Your Cervical Smear
KAREN EVENNETT

Overcoming Common Problems Series

Overcoming Common Problems Series

Is HRT Right for You?
DR ANNE MacGREGOR

Jealousy
DR PAUL HAUCK

Learning to Live with Multiple Sclerosis
DR ROBERT POVEY, ROBIN DOWIE
AND GILLIAN PRETT

Living with Angina
DR TOM SMITH

Living with Asthma
DR ROBERT YOUNGSON

Living with Diabetes
DR JOAN GOMEZ

Living with Grief
DR TONY LAKE

Living with High Blood Pressure
DR TOM SMITH

Making the Most of Yourself
GILL FOX AND SHEILA DAINOW

Menopause
RAEWYN MACKENZIE

The Migraine Diet Book
SUE DYSON

Motor Neurone Disease – A Family Affair
DR DAVID OLIVER

The Nervous Person's Companion
DR KENNETH HAMBLY

Out of Work – A Family Affair
ANNE LOVELL

Overcoming Anger
DR WINDY DRYDEN

Overcoming Guilt
DR WINDY DRYDEN

Overcoming Stress
DR VERNON COLEMAN

The Parkinson's Disease Handbook
DR RICHARD GODWIN-AUSTEN

The PMS Diet Book
KAREN EVENNETT

Serious Mental Illness – A Family Affair
GWEN HOWE

Subfertility Handbook, The
VIRGINIA IRONSIDE AND SARAH
BIGGS

Talking About Anorexia
How to cope with life without starving
MAROUSHKA MONRO

Ten Steps to Positive Living
DR WINDY DRYDEN

Think Your Way to Happiness
DR WINDY DRYDEN AND JACK
GORDON

**Understanding Obsessions and
Compulsions**
A self-help manual
DR FRANK TALLIS

Understanding Your Personality
Myers-Briggs and more
PATRICIA HEDGES

A Weight Off Your Mind
How to stop worrying about your body size
SUE DYSON

When your Child Comes Out
ANNE LOVELL

Overcoming Common Problems

Coping with Fibroids

Mary-Claire Mason

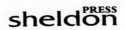

First published in Great Britain in 1997 by
Sheldon Press, SPCK, Marylebone Road, London NW1 4DU

British Library Cataloguing-in-Publication Data
A catalogue for this book is available from the British Library

ISBN 0–85969–766–5

Photoset by Deltatype Limited, Birkenhead, Merseyside
Printed in Great Britain by
Biddles Ltd, Guildford and Kings Lynn

Contents

Acknowledgements

I'd like to thank the doctors and complementary therapists who helped me with my research. I'm grateful in particular to Mr Chris Sutton, consultant gynaecologist at the Royal Surrey County Hospital, who so patiently and expertly answered all my questions at various points during my research. My thanks also to Mr Sutton's secretary Lynda Moorby, for her invaluable assistance. Also thanks to Mr Tony Parsons, consultant gynaecologist at the Hospital of St Cross, for his thoughts on fibroids. Finally I'd like to say a big thank-you to the women who shared their experiences with me, as these are central to this book.

Trademarks

The following trademarks are mentioned in this book:
Cyklokapron
Ponstan
Danol
Dimetriose
Panadol
Dicynene

1

Introduction

Many women know almost nothing about non-cancerous growths called fibroids which grow in the womb-wall. When I was asked to write an article about fibroids a couple of years ago, I realized just how ignorant I was about a condition which affects many women. Fibroids are common, particularly in women in their thirties and forties, and often occur at an earlier age in Afro-Caribbean women.

If you know nothing about fibroids it can be alarming to discover you have these lumps.

Angela's story

Angela was 30 when her fibroids were discovered six years ago. 'I felt so stupid, because I was a nurse but I didn't know anything about fibroids. I was scared stiff when the doctor told me after a routine examination that he thought I had fibroids. I became very upset because I thought they were cancerous growths. I cried and cried. I had further tests and was told I had a large fibroid and that my womb was the size of a 12-week to 16-week pregnancy. I thought: ''If it's that large, the cancer is too far gone''. After this I convinced myself that the medical staff were trying to hide something from me, even though they said there was nothing to worry about. It wasn't until I had the fibroid out and was told it was non-cancerous that I could believe I was safe.'

In fact, fibroids are very rarely cancerous – but Angela's worries are understandable and are shared by many women. This book looks at this issue, and at the other concerns which may arise if you are diagnosed as having fibroids.

Fibroids very often cause no problems at all – indeed, many women are unaware that they have fibroids. But these lumps can sometimes cause heavy periods, which may also be painful – as well as various other problems, including infertility and its accompanying heartache. The result can be much misery and ill-health. Yet in many women's health-books there is only a passing reference to fibroids.

1

Joan's story

Joan, a black woman in her mid-thirties, thinks her fibroids developed when she was in her late teens. 'I had very heavy periods, but I thought this was normal. In my early twenties I had to take time off work each month because I was so ill. I had awful cramps and nausea, and felt constantly tired. In order to cope with the heavy bleeding during my periods, I used to set my alarm clock for the middle of the night so I could change myself. If I didn't do this, the bedding would be soaked by morning. I also developed a pot-belly even though I was very fit. On one occasion I felt so awful that I had to go to Casualty. After a week of misdiagnosis, several fibroids were discovered – one was the size of an orange – and I had to have an operation to remove them. But the fibroids regrew and affected my fertility, so I had another operation to take them out. Shortly afterwards I became pregnant.' Joan now has two children and thinks she probably still has fibroids, but is untroubled by them at the moment.

In the past, women were usually advised to have a hysterectomy after a diagnosis of fibroids. Before the arrival of more sophisticated diagnostic techniques, there was no reliable way of knowing whether the fibroids might be cancerous, nor was there any way of distinguishing between fibroids and other conditions in that part of the body – such as ovarian cancer. Doctors therefore thought it best to open up the lower abdomen to see what was going on inside it, and then to remove the womb.

Sally's story

Ten years ago, at the age of 41, Sally was told she had fibroids after complaining that she felt bloated and full all the time. 'I was told I would have to have them out, and I only found out the day before the operation that the doctors were going to remove my womb. That was a bit of a shock. I wasn't offered any other sort of treatment.'

There is an awful lot that is still not known about fibroids, due to a lack of research into the subject. In the past, various assumptions were made about fibroids – assumptions which have not necessarily been backed up by any evidence. Today there is more interest in understanding why and how fibroids develop, and in offering women more treatment choices. Hysterectomy may still be the answer for some women – but with the latest diagnostic techniques, new drugs and surgical treatments, there are now other treatment options on offer.

As part of my research I talked both to women who have fibroids and to doctors with a special interest in the subject, as well as to non-conventional therapists. Various points emerged which are repeated throughout the book:

- little is still understood about fibroids and their natural development;
- fibroids often cause no trouble and need no treatment;
- fibroids can be wrongly blamed for causing problems – but depending on their size and position, fibroids can cause problems;
- there are various ways of coping with troublesome fibroids.

I've looked at current definitions of fibroids, and examined ideas about what causes these growths, how they are diagnosed and how, if you have symptom-producing fibroids, you can get the treatment that is right for you: two women with similar symptoms may want different treatments. I've looked at whether non-conventional therapies can help in any way. There is also a chapter devoted to self-help measures, which you may want to use alongside other treatments or which may in themselves be sufficient to help you cope with the problems which fibroids can cause.

2
What are fibroids?

Fibroids are tumours made up of smooth muscle-fibres which develop in the muscular wall of the womb (called the myometrium). You may be alarmed by the word tumour – but in fact fibroids are non-cancerous growths (with rare exceptions). Non-cancerous means they are self-contained, benign growths which do not have the ability to invade other body-tissue or spread around the body forming secondary growths. The lumps are made up of cells which have the same structure as normal womb-cells.

By contrast a cancer, sometimes called a malignant tumour, is made up of abnormal cells which divide more rapidly than the normal, surrounding cells. A malignant tumour differs from a benign tumour (such as a fibroid) in two ways:

1 As the cancer grows, it spreads and infiltrates surrounding tissue and may block passageways, destroy nerves and erode bone.
2 Cells from the cancer may spread, via the blood-system, to other parts of the body where they form secondary, malignant tumours.

If a fibroid is cancerous it's called a sarcoma, but this is very rare. It used to be thought that about one fibroid in 200 was cancerous – but the latest research suggests that only one fibroid in a thousand may be cancerous, and that these are usually found in women who have been through the menopause. The issue of whether or not fibroids can be cancerous does understandably concern women, and also has treatment implications; this is discussed in more detail in the next chapter.

It's useful to know the various medical names which are given to fibroids. A single fibroid is called myoma or fibromyoma, while several fibroids are called myomata or fibromyomata. Fibroids can also be called leiomyoma or leiomyomata.

Fibroids grow in the uterus – or womb, as it's commonly called – which is situated behind the bladder and in front of the intestines, in the pelvic cavity in the lower part of the abdomen.

The womb is a thick-walled organ which consists mainly of muscle. In a non-pregnant woman it is about 7.5–10 cm long and weighs about

60–90 g. It looks rather like an upside-down pear, and is a hollow muscle designed to hold the developing baby and then push it out at birth. In most women, the womb is angled slightly forwards to curve over the top of the bladder – though in some women, the womb is angled backwards towards the rectum. A broad ligament, like a double sheet of tissue, is attached to either side of the uterus. The womb is lined with a special material, the endometrium, a specialized tissue which prepares to receive the fertilized egg. The lining thickens and builds up each month under the influence of hormones from the ovaries. If there is no fertilized egg, the lining is shed each month during your period.

A fibroid is a cluster of small, spindle-shaped muscle-cells which grow within the muscular womb-wall at a faster rate than the surrounding cells. The fibroid is contained in a thick capsule or pouch which separates it from surrounding tissue. The fibroid may stay small or grow. Fibroids range in size: they can be as small as tiny seedlings or as big as large grapefruits and melons. The womb can become large and bulky, and you may look as though you are several months pregnant. Doctors actually talk about fibroid size by referring to the size of the womb during pregnancy, so for example you may be told your womb is the size of a 16-week pregnancy (which is quite large). You may just have one fibroid, but it's quite possible that you may have several or more fibroids. One doctor I spoke to had removed 107 fibroids from one woman – though the record number is 200.

Types of fibroids

Different types of fibroids grow in various parts of the womb-wall (see Figure 1). You may just have one type but could have a mix of various types.

- Submucous fibroids grow from under the womb-lining; they can grow on a stalk into the womb-cavity and sometimes come through the cervix (commonly called the neck of the womb) into the vagina. Estimates vary, but about five per cent of fibroids are thought to be submucous. Submucous fibroids on a stalk are sometimes called fibroid polyps.
- Intramural fibroids are perhaps the commonest ones; they form in

5

the middle of the womb-wall. According to one doctor, most women with this type of fibroid have a womb the size of an 8–12-week pregnancy.

- Subserous (also called sub-peritoneal) fibroids grow near the outer surface of the womb-wall, and can grow into the pelvic cavity, sometimes on a stalk. They can grow to an enormous size, and in exceptional cases can weigh as much as 15 kg or more.
- Cervical fibroids grow in the neck of the womb. This type of fibroid is uncommon, with only about two per cent of fibroids being in this position. It can be very tricky to remove a cervical fibroid if it's near to the ureters (the tubes which carry urine from the kidneys to the bladder).
- Intraligamentary fibroids occasionally form in the broad ligament, the sheet of tissue attached to either side of the womb.

Fibroids which grow on a stalk are referred to as *pedunculated*. A subserous fibroid on a stalk can occasionally become parasitic and attach itself to another organ in the pelvis, such as the bowel.

Who gets fibroids?

Lots of women have fibroids without being aware of their existence. This makes it difficult to estimate how common fibroids are – though some post-mortem studies have reported that as many as 75 per cent of women have fibroids. But the usual figures quoted are that fibroids occur in about one in five women over the age of 30, and one in three women over the age of 35 – though they can occur in women in their twenties. Afro-Caribbean women in particular are more likely to get fibroids in their twenties and even teens. Some studies also show that fibroids are three to nine times more common in black women. It's unclear how often fibroids occur in other racial groups. There's no information at the moment about whether more or fewer women are developing fibroids.

What causes fibroids?

It's important to say that nobody knows why fibroids develop – though there is a mixture of ideas about why fibroids grow at certain points during a woman's life. This lack of understanding has affected treatment choices.

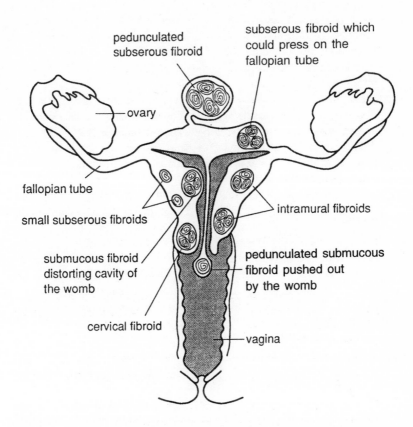

Figure 1 Places where fibroids can develop in the womb – few women would have them in all these areas.

Heredity does sometimes seem to play a part. If you have a close relative who has had fibroids you are more likely to have them. Twenty-nine-year-old Laura was diagnosed as having fibroids six years ago. Her grandmother, mother and maternal aunt have all had fibroids. The observation that fibroids are more common in black women also suggests that there is a genetic link.

Hormones

Though it's unclear why fibroids develop in the first place, there are ideas about what makes them grow. Fibroids are most often thought to be linked in some way to the female sex-hormone oestrogen, which is thought to make them grow. Progesterone (another sex-hormone) is thought to counteract this effect. Non-conventional therapists also often talk about a hormonal imbalance as causing fibroids.

A complex interplay of hormones controls the monthly menstrual cycle in which the egg is released. The hypothalamus, situated in the brain, has many functions – including control of hormonal systems throughout the body. It controls the pituitary gland, also situated in the brain, which in turn produces hormones essential for fertility. The two most important ones are FSH (follicle-stimulating hormone) and LH (luteinizing hormone), which prepare the ovaries for ovulation.

At the beginning of the menstrual cycle, FSH stimulates the ovaries to start producing an egg. As this happens, oestrogen released by the ovaries makes the womb-lining thicken in readiness for a possible pregnancy. This is known as the proliferative or follicular phase. The pituitary gland then produces LH which triggers the release of the egg. The corpus luteum, which forms after ovulation, produces progesterone, often called the pregnancy hormone. This makes the womb-lining swollen and thick. These changes occur during the second part of the cycle, which is known as the secretory or luteal phase. So hormonal levels change during the monthly cycle, with oestrogen-levels peaking when the egg is released at ovulation, and progesterone-levels peaking during the second part of the cycle.

There are various types of oestrogen in the body: oestradiol, oestriol and oestrone. Oestradiol is the most powerful of these, and is most abundant before the menopause. In post-menopausal women, oestrone is the main type of oestrogen. The main type of oestrogen during pregnancy is oestriol.

Oestradiol is the type of oestrogen which is thought to be linked to fibroid growth – though it's not thought to cause fibroids to develop in the first place. This theory has been developed by researchers looking at who gets fibroids and what happens to fibroids during pregnancy and after the menopause.

Oestrogen and fibroids

In 1986 a study was published by the Oxford Family Planning Association (FPA) which provided some information about the women who have fibroids. The study included only white women, so it's unclear what relevance the findings have for other racial groups. These findings, plus doctors' observations about how fibroids grow at certain points in a woman's life, led to the development of the oestrogen theory.

- Thin women seem less likely to get fibroids. In the FPA study, women who weighed more than 70 kg were three times more likely to have fibroids than women who weighed less than 50 kg. The analysis took account of both height and weight. Oestrogen was implicated because overweight women produce more oestrogen from fatty tissue. However, thin women can have fibroids – in fact, I spoke to one woman who suffers from being underweight and who, during a routine examination, was recently diagnosed as having fibroids. But the lumps were causing her no problems.
- Women who haven't had children seem at greater risk. The FPA study, for example, found that women who had been through five pregnancies had only a quarter the risk of women who hadn't ever been pregnant. This observation led to the idea that women who go through fewer pregnancies, or never have children, are more susceptible to developing fibroids. One possible explanation for this is that though oestrogen levels are high in pregnancy the main type of oestrogen is not the powerful oestradiol but oestriol – which is less potent. On the other hand, existing fibroids sometimes go through a growth spurt during pregnancy, which seems to contradict this theory. It's also not clear that pregnancy does protect against fibroids. Low family-size may be a consequence and not a cause of fibroids. So some women may find it more difficult to get pregnant because they have fibroids.
- The FPA study found that women who had been on the combined contraceptive Pill for ten years had a significantly lower risk of

9

having fibroids. The brands of Pill that contained higher amounts of progestogen (a synthetic form of progesterone) were most protective. It's thought that the progestogen in the Pill counteracts the effects of oestrogen. A more recent study in 1995 in the *British Journal of Obstetrics and Gynaecology* also reported that the Pill had some sort of protective effect.

• The Pill may also be protective for another reason. Some doctors think that, in the normal cycle, the peak-level of oestrogen at ovulation may be linked to fibroids. So you may be protected if you take the type of combined Pill which gives you the same dose of hormones each day during the artificial cycle. There have also been fears in the past that the Pill could make fibroids grow – but this was at a time when the Pill contained higher amounts of oestrogen.

• Some doctors think that anovulatory cycles, in which no egg is released, are linked to fibroid development. Anovulatory cycles are more common in women coming up to the menopause, and may also be linked to stress. In these cycles, only oestrogen is released – and though it's not clear how much oestrogen is released in these types of cycles one point is clear. There is no release of progesterone because ovulation does not occur. It's claimed therefore that *oestrogen dominance* makes fibroid growth more likely because there is no progesterone to offset the effects of oestrogen.

• Women who smoke appear to be less likely to develop fibroids. The explanation for this is that smoking reduces oestrogen levels.

• It's generally accepted that fibroids normally shrink after the menopause, and it's thought that this happens because of the decline in oestrogen-levels after the menopause.

• Fibroids sometimes start to grow again when women take oestrogen in the form of HRT (hormone replacement therapy) after the menopause.

Discussion

The main explanation of the cause of fibroids is that oestrogen is linked in some way to fibroid growth – but as we have seen, the evidence about risk factors is unclear to say the least. Until recently progesterone was thought to offset the effects of oestrogen. For example, as we have seen, brands of contraceptive Pill containing higher amounts of progestogen are thought to be protective.

The question of how hormones influence fibroids is a complex one.

It's important to emphasize again that very little is still understood about the link. But some researchers now think that not only oestrogen but also progesterone may promote fibroid growth – an observation which makes some sense given that the two hormones are so interlinked.

A paper in the *British Journal of Obstetrics and Gynaecology* in November 1993 – called 'The regulation of fibroid growth: time for a re-think?' – called for a re-examination of the idea that oestrogen stimulates fibroid growth and progesterone prevents it, in the hope of this leading to improved drug-treatments. According to the paper, there was evidence that progesterone might be implicated: for example, in one study a drug which reduced the effects of progestogen in the body inhibited fibroid growth.

A research paper published in January 1995 in the *American Journal of Obstetrics and Gynaecology* (called 'Progesterone: A critical role in the pathogenesis of uterine myomas') reviewed various studies. In one study, progestogen was used to treat fibroids. Contrary to what might be expected, womb-size increased during treatment and reduced once treatment had stopped. In a more recent study of women with troublesome fibroids, the growths reduced in size when the women were given a drug which stopped their ovaries producing oestrogen. But when they were then given progestogen as well as the original drug, the fibroids seemed to increase in size. The researchers concluded that progestogen reduced the effectiveness of treatment – and that more research must be done into the effects of different types of progestogens and progesterone on fibroid growth.

But some doctors are sceptical, saying that the various research findings need to be critically examined. It could be, for example, that some of the progestogen drugs make fibroids swell rather than grow.

However, researchers who support the idea that progesterone could stimulate fibroid growth make several points. It may be that the drugs which shut down the ovaries are successful not only because they stop oestrogen production but also progesterone production. Progesterone-levels are also higher in pregnancy, which may explain why fibroids sometimes grow at this time. Fibroids may shrink after the menopause not only because oestrogen production declines but because progesterone is no longer produced.

So both hormones may well play some part in triggering fibroid growth – though quite how is not currently understood. Some researchers think that the sharp rise and fall of the two hormones during normal cycles may be to blame. This may explain why the type of combined contraceptive Pill which gives the same hormonal dose each day might be protective. Fibroids also seem to be linked to abnormal amounts of growth-factors – proteins which stimulate cell growth. Other ideas about what causes fibroid growth come from non-conventional therapists, who tend to talk about the body being out of balance. These ideas are considered in Chapter 9.

Prevention

Since it's unclear what causes fibroids, it's difficult to know how to prevent them developing. But two points emerge from the FPA study which are worth thinking about if you know that fibroids run in your family and you want to try and reduce your chance of developing them.

- Findings indicate that fibroids are more common in women who weigh over 70 kg – so it makes sense to keep your weight under control. If it turns out that there is no connection between weight and fibroid development, it still makes sense to keep your weight under control for your health generally.
- The combined Pill may be protective, so if you need a contraceptive method you may want to discuss with your doctor whether the Pill is suitable for you. There's more information on the Pill in Chapter 6.

A more pressing question if you already have fibroids is what can you do to stop them becoming troublesome? Most doctors would say there is little you can do. But some non-conventional therapists talk about the importance of getting the body into balance and reducing stress levels to improve hormonal balance. There are also various ways of helping yourself, as discussed in Chapter 10. Finally, it's also important to note that fibroids do not inevitably become increasingly troublesome.

Summary

Fibroids are commonplace and there are different types of fibroids. It's unclear why they develop, but conventional ideas about why fibroids increase in size are starting to be re-examined. This in turn may lead to improved drug-treatments.

3

What problems do fibroids cause?

In the past, fibroids were often removed on the grounds that they were potentially dangerous. I spoke to one researcher who was keen to correct this idea. She went to the other extreme and said that fibroids are a normal part of a woman's make-up, do not cause medical problems and are a nuisance at worst.

It's true that fibroids are not life-threatening (except in rare cases), and often cause no problems.

Lesley's story

> Eighteen years ago, at the age of 33, Lesley was told she had fibroids during a routine internal examination. 'I was very upset because I'd never heard about fibroids. I was just about to get married and I was desperately worried that the fibroids might affect my chances of getting pregnant. In fact, I had no problems conceiving and had a normal pregnancy and birth. I then had another child and again had no problems. I'm now 51 and still have the fibroids – but I've never had any trouble with them apart from the fact that my stomach is quite large.'

But research suggests that perhaps half of the women with fibroids do experience symptoms, sometimes distressing ones, as a result of having fibroids. Some women put up with the symptoms, not realizing that they are due to fibroids. Whether or not you have problems will depend on the size, number and location of fibroids in the womb-wall. The good news is that fibroids normally shrink and become less troublesome after the menopause – it's thought that this is due to changes in hormone-production.

It is best to divide problems into two broad groups:

1 The symptoms which suggest that you may have troublesome fibroids.
2 The issues or problems that can be caused by fibroids.

Symptoms

Heavy and sometimes painful periods

Fibroids in themselves are not painful, except in certain circumstances (see the section, 'Painful fibroids', later in this chapter). But fibroids can cause distressing symptoms, perhaps the most common one being heavy and sometimes painful periods. Many of the women I spoke to mentioned these symptoms – such as passing large liver-like clots, as well as flooding (a sudden downpour of blood). The bleeding and pain can disrupt sleep, leaving women exhausted and depressed. Normal life can be seriously disrupted.

Rachel's story

Rachel, aged 40, recalls: 'I'd had heavy periods for a long time – ever since my late twenties – but I thought this was normal. For the first two days of my period I used to flood, and needed to go to the toilet every half-hour or so to change my sanitary protection. It was usual for me to soil the bed several times a night, and I couldn't go away or accept invitations to stay in other people's houses during my period. I was very embarrassed by the flooding, but could only talk to my closest friends about what was happening.'

Sarah's story

Fifty-two-year-old Sarah started having heavy periods when she was 37, after the birth of her second child. 'My periods lasted five days, but the second and third days were very heavy and also painful. I used to pass great clots like lumps of liver. I didn't do anything about this because I could manage the bleeding. I knew how long it would last, and that it would stop and I would have a chance to recover. There were occasional problems. One day, for example, I couldn't leave the office because I was bleeding so badly. My periods were heavy for about three years, then they improved – but when I was in my late forties the heavy bleeding started up again and was very difficult to control.'

Joanna's story

Joanna, 37, recalls: 'About seven years ago my periods started to get really heavy and prolonged, lasting about ten days. I used to carry stacks of night-time towels in my handbag, and had to change every two hours or so at work. Tampons and daytime towels were hopelessly inadequate.'

Louise's story

Louise, 40, had fibroids removed when she was 29. Last year she started having period problems again, and was told that her fibroids had returned. 'I had incredibly bad cramps and was bleeding all the time. I had to wear incontinence pads to cope with the flow. It was very embarrassing because on one occasion I was sitting down at work when I started flooding.'

Fibroids are a common cause of heavy bleeding. It can be difficult knowing exactly what is meant by this term and, like Rachel, many women accept their bleeding-pattern as normal. But it is possible for medical professionals to measure blood-loss by analysing used sanitary protection. The definition of menorrhagia (the medical term for heavy bleeding) is blood-loss of over 80 ml during a period (80 ml is about a small teacupful). On average, women lose about 30–40 ml each period. Women can have heavy periods for a number of reasons but some research suggests that blood-loss is particularly heavy in women who have fibroids. In one study, 40 per cent of women who were losing more than 200 ml each period had fibroids. Blood-loss can sometimes be torrential – for example, one woman lost a litre a month.

There are various theories about why fibroids cause problems – though there is still some uncertainty about the exact role that fibroids play in heavy bleeding. I spoke to one woman who thought that the fibroids themselves bled during her period. But fibroids do not actually bleed during menstruation – though they can bleed in other circumstances (see the section, 'Degeneration', later in this chapter). But they are linked to heavy menstrual blood-flow for a number of reasons.

- Submucous fibroids are commonly blamed for causing heavy bleeding as they can increase the area of womb-lining by perhaps 10 to 15 times – so there is far more lining to shed each month. But some researchers now think that submucous fibroids are not always to blame, and that fibroids in other positions can also increase flow.

15

- Fibroids may interfere with clotting mechanisms, making it difficult for the bleeding to stop.
- There are more blood-vessels in the womb-wall because of the growths, and this increases the likelihood of heavy bleeding. So just treating submucous fibroids may not be effective in reducing blood-loss if you also have other sorts of fibroids.
- Clots are often passed. Substances in the womb-lining normally stop clots forming so that the blood can flow easily from the womb. But during heavy bleeding, these anti-clotting agents get used up and then the blood starts to clot.

Lucy's story

Lucy was 36 when she first started passing clots. 'I suddenly started having very heavy periods and passing big lumps of stuff. I was very frightened and rushed off to my doctor who diagnosed fibroids.'

You may find you have a lot of pain during your period. The clots can sometimes cause pain as they pass through the neck of the womb, particularly in women who have never had children. If a submucous fibroid grows into the womb-cavity on a stalk, the womb may try to push it out through the cervix, causing cramping pains. Periods can also become irregular and you may have spotting in between periods – though these two symptoms are less common.

It's important to emphasize that fibroids may not be the cause of heavy bleeding. Other conditions which can cause heavy periods include ovarian cysts, hormonal imbalance and changes particularly in the years coming up to the menopause, endometriosis, underactive thyroid, pelvic infection and blood-clotting disorders. In about 50 per cent of cases, no cause can be found for heavy bleeding. It is often difficult to know what's causing bleeding problems.

Joanna's story

Joanna, 53, is approaching the menopause and has been told she has a fibroid the size of a golf-ball. At the moment her periods are unpredictable and sometimes very heavy. 'I became very frightened when I bled solidly for two days. I just had to lie down during that time.' Joanna isn't clear whether the fibroid is responsible for the bleeding or whether it's due to changing hormone-levels in her body as she approaches the menopause.

Anaemia

Very heavy periods can sometimes – but not always – cause anaemia. Many women carry on struggling with work and home life unaware they have this condition.

Susan's story

Susan found out she was severely anaemic. She had been putting up with very heavy periods for some years. 'I had been bleeding very heavily for a few days and was having non-stop flooding and passing huge clots. One day at work I suddenly found I had no energy. I could hardly walk across the floor. I managed to get through the day and dragged myself home, where I collapsed. I saw my doctor the next day and had a blood-test done. The results showed I was extremely anaemic and I ended up having a blood transfusion.

Anaemia is a condition in which the concentration of the oxygen-carrying pigment in the blood (called haemoglobin) is below normal. Haemoglobin molecules are carried inside red blood-cells, and take oxygen from the lungs to body-tissue. Iron is an essential part of haemoglobin – and iron-deficiency anaemia is the most common form. Women are particularly prone to this type of anaemia, which affects about one in twenty women, because heavy bleeding reduces the amount of iron.

A woman's normal haemoglobin-levels are 11.5 g–16 g per 100 ml of blood. Below 10 g you may feel headachy, tired and lethargic. Below 8 g, watch out for dizziness (due to less oxygen reaching the brain), angina, chest-pains (due to reduced oxygen supply to the heart) and palpitations as the heart has to work harder. If you're anaemic you may need a blood transfusion before you have an operation to remove fibroids.

Warnings signs of anaemia include: tiredness, headaches, pallor, dizziness, weakness, rapid pulse, palpitations, sore tongue. Treatments and self-help measures for anaemia are covered in Chapter 10.

Pressure symptoms

Fibroids can become quite large, yet cause no obvious symptoms. But sometimes a bulky womb can press on surrounding organs and cause a number of symptoms which you may not realize are due to fibroids.

Mary's story

Mary, 59, had her womb removed a year ago because she had been having slight post-menopausal bleeding. When her womb was removed it was the size of a 20-week pregnancy and had a large subserous fibroid attached to it. 'I never knew I had it. The only symptom was a bit of bladder frequency but it wasn't really a problem.'

Helen's story

Helen's fibroids were responsible for a large stomach. 'I was very fit in my early twenties but I had this big belly – I never understood what caused it until the fibroids were discovered.'

Lucy's story

Lucy has had several pressure symptoms: 'I have a bit of a pot-belly. More recently I've started having to go to the loo every hour at work, which is a bit awkward – and I get up perhaps three times a night. Sex is also mildly uncomfortable because I think one of the fibroids is pressing on my vagina.'

Ruth's story

Ruth, 51, has just had her fibroid taken out. 'The fibroid was diagnosed when I was in my mid-forties. I was a bit bloated and was going to the loo more and more. The doctor said no treatment was needed, but decided that the fibroid should be monitored. Over the next few years it gradually became bigger until it was huge, the size of a melon. I was told my womb was the size of a 19-week pregnancy. My stomach was massive and I could actually feel the fibroid through my abdomen. By now I was having to go to the loo all the time, but I didn't have any other symptoms and felt fine. However, as I was having to spend all my time in the loo, I couldn't lead a normal life.'

Whether or not fibroids cause pressure symptoms depends on their size and location – for instance, whether they are on the front or back of the womb. An enlarged womb can press on the bladder or bowel causing various symptoms. It's estimated that about five per cent of fibroids cause various types of bladder problems. Cervical fibroids, in particular, may make passing urine more difficult. Urinary symptoms include wanting to pass urine frequently, maybe having to strain to do so initially. There is also a risk of developing cystitis from stagnant urine in the bladder which becomes infected. It may occasionally be impossible to pass water. This is a serious problem and requires urgent hospital treatment, in which a tube is put into the bladder to empty it. Cervical fibroids can very occasionally put pressure on the ureters, causing kidney damage. A fibroid pressing on the bowel may cause constipation or haemorrhoids, though this is uncommon.

Summary of pressure and related symptoms

- Pressure on other organs can sometimes cause various symptoms, including pelvic discomfort (sometimes described as a sense of fullness with a dragging sensation), constipation, varicose veins (if fibroids press on veins from the legs).
- Changes in bladder and bowel habits.
- A persistent, dull back-ache. This may happen for several reasons. The fibroid may pull the womb backwards slightly, which can sometimes cause discomfort. The fibroids can cause a build-up of fluid in the pelvis, which is uncomfortable.
- Painful love-making. Fibroids can cause discomfort during love-making, depending on where the fibroids are positioned. If a bulky womb or subserous fibroid presses against an ovary, it could cause pain during deep penetration. It can also be painful making love if a fibroid presses on the neck of the womb or starts coming through into the vagina. This may result in bleeding during love-making, and sometimes in spotting and cramping between periods.
- A cervical fibroid can sometimes cause inflammation in the neck of the womb, which may result in a discharge.

It's important to see your doctor if you have any of these symptoms to find out what's causing the problem. It could be fibroids or some other condition.

Painful fibroids

Fibroids are not normally painful but they can be in certain circumstances.

Torsion

A large fibroid on a stalk can twist, cutting off its own blood-supply. Torsion, as it's called, can be very painful. Symptoms include shock, vomiting, low abdominal pain and fever. The symptoms may initially indicate an ovarian cyst which has twisted. The fibroid may need to be removed, but you may just need to rest and take painkillers.

This condition does not always cause severe pain and the fibroid may die away of its own accord. One expert commented that it's rare for fibroids to twist as most aren't on a stalk.

Fibroids can also be painful if they degenerate during pregnancy (see the pregnancy section below).

Degeneration

Degeneration is a general term for the physical and chemical changes in tissue. Degeneration is a feature of ageing, and may be due to various things – including reduced blood-supply. Parts of the fibroid can start to shrink if it doesn't receive enough blood. There's no research into which fibroids are most likely to degenerate, but anecdotal evidence suggests that large fibroids are more likely to do so. Various types of degeneration occur frequently, but are usually not a problem. (Red degeneration is covered below, in the section on pregnancy.)

After the menopause, fibroids typically shrink due to changing hormone-levels. In older women it's quite common to find womb-stones. These are fibroids which have become calcified and bone-like, and which show up on X-rays.

Problems

Apart from period problems and pressure problems, fibroids can cause other potential problems.

In pregnancy

Red degeneration

Red degeneration occurs during pregnancy, when fibroids may grow rapidly due to increased hormone-levels. The fibroid swells, becomes red, softens and starts to die. There is acute pain because the blood-supply cannot always get to the centre of the growth.

Red degeneration can make the womb contract, risking early labour or miscarriage. If this happens and you have cramping pains, tell your doctor. You would be admitted to hospital and the diagnosis confirmed by ultrasound scan, a diagnostic technique described in Chapter 4.

Drugs are given to relieve the pain and stop the womb cramping – but symptoms usually resolve of their own accord.

There is contradictory evidence about how often red degeneration occurs in pregnancy. About two per cent of pregnancies occur in women with fibroids, according to one study. But only one in 10 of these women experience problems, usually red degeneration as a result of having fibroids. However, another study reported that about a half of pregnant patients with fibroids suffered red degeneration. Yet another study used ultrasound to monitor fibroid growth throughout pregnancy. The results showed that only a tiny number of fibroids grew during pregnancy, usually during the first three months, and that they then stopped growing or even got smaller during the later part of pregnancy.

Women with fibroids are warned about the possibility of red degeneration occurring in pregnancy, one specialist stated. In her experience this usually happens in the middle weeks of pregnancy. But she emphasized that it's not dangerous, does not usually endanger the pregnancy and gets better on its own.

Other pregnancy problems

Other fibroid-related problems in pregnancy are an increased risk of premature labour and a higher miscarriage rate (perhaps two to three times greater than normal). A very large fibroid in the womb may interfere occasionally with childbirth, especially if it's near the neck of the womb. In order to prevent problems, a Caesarean may be recommended.

If you have fibroids and are thinking of getting pregnant, it's worth talking to your doctor about whether you should have the fibroids removed before you conceive. This will depend on their size and location – as well as on the doctor's views.

Some doctors think that the removal of fibroids before conception may be advisable, but others do not. One expert said that, as fibroids do not usually cause significant problems during pregnancy, you would not be advised to have your fibroids removed just because you were planning to get pregnant. Surgery carries risks – and can also sometimes cause infertility if it results in scarring or infection in the abdomen. However, if a woman has had previous pregnancy complications due to fibroids, it may make sense to remove the growths before she gets pregnant. (See also the next section on infertility.)

Helen's story

Helen has been through two pregnancies. 'The doctors were worried about what would happen to the fibroids, but though they started growing in the early weeks of my pregnancy, they stabilized. I had no other problems. I was given a Caesarean just in case of potential difficulties, as the fibroids were round the neck of the womb. At the six-week check-up after the birth of my baby, I was told I still had the fibroids and not to leave it too long if I wanted another baby. I conceived straightaway, and had an uneventful pregnancy and then another Caesarean.'

Infertility

The idea that fibroids can cause infertility is subject to debate. Some experts argue that fibroids do not cause problems because many women of childbearing age have fibroids and get pregnant with no apparent difficulty. But other doctors and researchers disagree – and so did some of the women I spoke to.

Laura's story

This uncertainty is reflected in Laura's story. Aged 29, she became pregnant for the first time six years ago. 'At seven weeks I miscarried. The doctor scrapped my womb out afterwards to make sure nothing was left inside. It was at this point he discovered I had fibroids, and said I would need to have them taken out. We were in the process of moving to another area, so I didn't do anything until we had settled into our new home. I then went to the local hospital and was told that the fibroids were nothing to worry about, and just to wait and see.

'Over the next year I tried unsuccessfully to get pregnant. Meanwhile my periods were getting heavier and more painful, sometimes lasting up to 14 days. I was passing saucer-shaped clots, flooding and getting very tired. Our sex-life suffered because of all this. I decided to see a doctor about my infertility. Some tests were done and I was told that one of my tubes was blocked. They discovered fibroids inside the womb and decided to remove them through my vagina – but the operation was stopped because the surgeon decided it was too difficult. I was then referred to a doctor who was supposed to be an expert in removing fibroids, but he eventually decided it was too dangerous to remove them.

'I then went through two IVF attempts to get pregnant. In desperation, I went to another fertility specialist who initially wasn't concerned about the fibroids. He said I wasn't ovulating properly, so he dealt with this problem first. But last year he did some more tests which showed that the fibroids were distorting the inside of my womb. I think this was making it difficult for the baby to implant properly in the womb-lining. This makes sense, as I felt at one point that I had conceived but nothing happened. So the specialist decided to remove the fibroids, which he thought were responsible for my problems. Apparently I had them all over the place. Eight lemon-sized lumps were removed. One on the front of my womb had gone from the outside through to the inside of my womb. I was told it looked like a ball stuck in a tennis racket. That was a year ago and everything seems to have healed up – but I'm still not pregnant. But my periods are much lighter now, and my womb is about the size of a 10-week pregnancy. At one point it was huge, about the size of a 24-week pregnancy. The whole business has been exhausting and draining. We've been given so much conflicting information and lost valuable time as a result.'

Joanna's story

Joanna tried for a baby unsuccessfully seven years ago. 'I went for some investigations at my local hospital and fibroids were diagnosed. I don't know exactly where the fibroids were, but they were large and had apparently made my womb a very strange shape. But I was told the fibroids were not responsible for my infertility.

'I had various other investigations, and was then put on fertility drugs. They couldn't find much wrong and said we had unexplained infertility. I wasn't happy with this diagnosis, so I went to a specialist fertility clinic. More checks were done. A special dye was put into my womb and an X-ray done which showed that my womb was very distorted. It was three times the size it should be and the womb-wall was bulging inwards. The procedure was a bit uncomfortable but it was worth it. The infertility specialist thought the fibroids might be causing problems, and recommended that I had them removed. I had an operation, and two were removed – one the size of an orange. Six weeks after the operation I saw the consultant who said it was fine to try for a baby, and a couple of months later I conceived and had a normal pregnancy. I've concluded that the fibroids were definitely to blame. If I hadn't done my own research I might never have had any children.'

Lucy's story

Lucy was told that her fibroids, one of which was on the outside of her womb, wouldn't interfere with her fertility. 'I was 36 then and hoping I could have children. But I never got pregnant. I'm 50 now, and it's too late to have children. I suspect the fibroids may in some way have affected my fertility.'

Joan's story

Joan had fertility problems before she conceived her first baby. 'I had fibroids all over my womb. I had the latest surgical techniques to remove the biggest ones which were making me infertile, and also those which were making my periods painful and heavy. Afterwards I was monitored closely, because the remaining fibroids were growing. A few months later I became pregnant. I've now got two children and the fibroids aren't troubling me at the moment. But it's possible I may have to see the surgeon again about having some fibroids removed if I want a third child.'

The question of whether fibroids can affect fertility again depends on their size and location. About one in six couples experiences problems getting pregnant. Between 2 and 10 per cent of these couples may have fertility problems due to fibroids – and the figure could be higher if the woman is black.

There are various ideas about why fibroids might affect fertility. If fibroids distort the womb-cavity they may prevent the embryo from implanting in the womb-lining. Subserous fibroids may press on the Fallopian tubes making it more difficult for the egg to move down the tube. Large fibroids may interfere with the womb-contractions which help sperm move towards the egg. It's also possible that large fibroids interfere with the growth of the embryo, and encourage early miscarriage. It's important to talk to a fertility specialist about what should be done if there is evidence that fibroids are distorting the inside of the womb or pressing on the Fallopian tubes.

It's also important to get a proper diagnosis if you are having problems getting pregnant. Conception is a matter of chance, even for couples of normal fertility – and some have more luck than others. After six months of trying, only six out of ten couples will have conceived. The general rule is to try for a year and then see your doctor. You can extend this to 18 months if you are under 30, when fertility is higher and reduce it to six months if you're over 35, when fertility starts to decline. But go straightaway if you have heavy or painful periods, or any of the other fibroid symptoms.

If possible, try and go to a specialist fertility clinic for tests and investigations. Joanna thought the advice she received from her local hospital was not up-to-date. The self-help groups listed at the back of the book can provide information on how to choose a clinic.

Cancer

One question which worries many women is whether fibroids can become cancerous. The latest evidence suggests that malignant degeneration – that is, when a benign tumour turns into a malignant one – is very rare: less than one fibroid in a thousand is cancerous. And it's unclear why a fibroid becomes cancerous. It may be that a particular fibroid is predisposed to cancerous changes and that four or five factors trigger the changes. It may also be that fibroids don't become cancerous, but that the tumour is malignant from the outset – there are apparently no studies which show fibroids becoming cancerous. There is no evidence at the moment as to whether certain risk factors make you more likely to have malignant fibroids. Cancerous fibroids occur mainly in post-menopausal women.

Nowadays doctors do not remove fibroids because of worries that the growths may become cancerous – unless there are good reasons to do so. There may be warning signs, or an ultrasound scan may show up suspicious-looking growths – though other types of degeneration can sometimes look suspicious. Warnings signs include:

- Post-menopausal bleeding.
- Fibroid growth after the menopause.
- Irregular vaginal bleeding.
- Rapid fibroid growth. However, little is known about the natural life-history of fibroids, and benign fibroids can also go through growth-spurts.
- Large fibroids are thought more likely to be cancerous. However

there are apparently no studies which show that you are more at risk of having a malignant fibroid if you have large fibroids.

- Certain hormonal drugs make fibroids shrink for a time; if a fibroid does not shrink, it may be cancerous.

If you have these sorts of symptoms, the doctor will want to do various tests to check not only for the rare possibility of a malignant fibroid, but also for other cancers (such as cancer of the womb-lining). (See Chapter 4 for details of diagnostic tests.) If the fibroid is clearly cancerous, the doctor will want to remove the whole womb. Chapter 8 deals with the different types of hysterectomy.

Termination of pregnancy

Is an abortion more painful if you have fibroids? There do not seem to be any studies on this – but one woman wrote to *Women's Health* about her abortion when she was 12 weeks pregnant. She was warned to expect pain because she had large fibroids. This happened, and she had to stay in bed for a couple of weeks afterwards because of awful cramping pains.

One doctor explained to me that if you have fibroids, there is a slightly increased complication rate because it can be more difficult to empty the womb properly. There may also be some bleeding problems after the procedure, because the womb does not close so well. Due to changes in the blood-supply, there may also be degenerative changes in the fibroids which can cause discomfort. But there aren't any major problems. If you know you have fibroids, discuss this with the doctor beforehand.

Other gynaecological conditions

It's important to be aware of other conditions in the pelvic region. You may have fibroids as well as some of these other conditions, and this may complicate matters. It's possible that fibroids may be blamed for symptoms caused by these other conditions. It's also possible that one of these other conditions could be mistakenly diagnosed as fibroids. However, with the latest diagnostic techniques, discussed in Chapter 4, it's now much easier to get an accurate diagnosis. If you have co-existing conditions, then any treatment plan needs to take account of this.

Ovarian problems

Doctors are always anxious to check that the ovaries are not cancerous as the outlook for ovarian cancer is often poor. The two ovaries are situated one either side of the womb immediately below the opening of the Fallopian tubes. Each ovary, shaped like an almond, is about 3 cm long and 2 cm wide and contains lots of cavities called follicles in which egg-cells develop.

Ovarian cysts

Ovarian cysts are common, and 95 per cent of them are non-cancerous. There are various types of ovarian cysts, but the most common ones – called functional cysts – are linked to the monthly cycle. The follicle which releases the egg fills with fluid rather than breaking down in the normal way.

Functional cysts may cause no problems, particularly if they are small; but they can cause abdominal discomfort and start to press on other organs if they enlarge. Some can grow to the size of a tennis ball and weigh a lot. Most disappear without treatment. The ovary may have to be removed; though it is sometimes possible just to remove the cyst.

The symptoms can be very similar to those of fibroids. For example, swelling, abdominal discomfort (though this tends to be one-sided), pain during love-making, heavy or painful periods. If pain starts in the second part of your cycle, is one-sided and lasts through to your period, you may have an ovarian cyst. You may have severe pain, nausea and fever if the cyst twists or ruptures. Large cysts are big enough to feel in the abdomen, and can be mistaken for middle-aged spread. Cysts can enlarge rapidly without causing symptoms, and may not be diagnosed until they are very large. They can also cause pressure symptoms, such as needing to pass water more frequently, and constipation.

Diana's story

Diana's fibroids were discovered ten years ago, when she was 36. A year or so later the diagnosis was confirmed by another doctor, who also said that Diana had an ovarian cyst. 'I'd never had any significant problems with the fibroids or cysts at that point – but a couple of years later I had an operation to remove the fibroids. The fibroids regrew, but didn't cause any problems. But a couple of years ago I had the most excruciating pain in my abdomen. A cyst was found on my right ovary, which was removed. I then kept having problems with cysts on the left ovary, which had to be drained. The fibroids weren't a problem, apart from causing a bulky womb; but in the end I had to have the other ovary out, and it seemed sensible to have my womb taken out at the same time.'

Sarah's story

Sarah was having very heavy, painful periods in her late forties. 'My periods were getting longer and heavier, and I had bleeding in between periods. I also sometimes had acute pain on one side, like a screwdriver twisting inside me. I eventually had an ultrasound scan, and they found I had fibroids as well as an ovarian cyst. The gynaecologist was keen on taking my womb and ovaries out as she was worried about the possibility of ovarian cancer developing – but I'm not prepared to have this done as I don't think there is any evidence of cancer.'

Ovarian cancer

This can occur at any age, but is most common after the age of 50. It is the most deadly of all the gynaecological cancers because it's not usually detected until it's widespread, when treatments are less effective. Each year 5,000 cases are diagnosed, but the outlook is very poor for most sufferers. It is sometimes possible for the cancer to become fixed to the womb so that it can be confused with a fibroid. But the cancer looks different and grows rapidly. Treatment consists of removing the ovaries, the Fallopian tubes and the womb, followed by courses of anti-cancer drugs.

Symptoms of ovarian cancer are vague and include abdominal discomfort and swelling, bouts of constipation and diarrhoea, nausea, abnormal vaginal bleeding. The abdomen sometimes swells up with fluid. Pain is rare.

Endometriosis

Endometriosis is a condition in which the lining of the womb gets into other parts of the body, usually the pelvic cavity. It's most common in women aged 25–40, and it's unclear what causes it. The womb-lining elsewhere in the body responds to the normal monthly cycle, and bleeds into surrounding tissue. This inappropriate bleeding can produce cysts, and cause inflammation and scarring in tissue. Cysts often form on the ovaries, lined with cells which bleed during menstruation.

Endometriosis produces a variety of symptoms again similar to those of fibroids; but diagnostic techniques can distinguish between the two conditions. Key symptoms include painful and heavy periods, painful love-making, infertility, swollen abdomen, bowel and bladder problems, back pain. Treatment depends on the severity of symptoms. Hormonal drugs may be given to shrink the endometrial patches, or surgery used to remove the tissue. If this doesn't help and you have severe symptoms, your doctor may suggest a hysterectomy.

Adenomyosis

Adenomyosis is a little-understood condition, which has been recognized for over a 120 years. Deposits from the womb-lining are found in the muscular womb-wall. It's more unusual to get a big nodule, called an adenomyoma, which resembles a fibroid. But these nodules are not encased in a capsule and unlike fibroids cannot be shelled out.

It tends to affect women in their forties. It may cause problems by interfering with normal womb-contractions, affecting the ability of blood-vessels to close during periods. Classic symptoms include heavy periods, pain, and sometimes abdominal swelling – so it can be confused with fibroids initially. But many women have no symptoms. The condition is treated with hormones, which are used to shrink the tissue.

Summary

Fibroids often cause no problems at all, and usually shrink after the menopause. But they can cause a range of problems. Symptoms to look out for include:

- Heavy periods – if you have to start using more sanitary protection than you used to, or if you have to use a tampon and pad together, or several pads.
- Passing clots.
- Your periods lasting longer than previously.

- Pain during your periods. It may be intense or dull and aching.
- A full, heavy, dragging feeling in your lower abdomen. A sense of fullness.
- Having to pass water more often, or changing bowel habits.
- Anaemia symptoms, such as weakness and tiredness.
- Having difficulty getting pregnant.

4

Diagnosis

You may actually be able to feel a lump in your abdomen, but often there are no obvious symptoms of fibroids. They may be detected during routine check-ups – for example, if you are having a cervical smear or when you are pregnant. Don't be alarmed if this happens.

Susan's story

Susan had no fibroid symptoms, but was having a routine internal examination. 'I was a bit alarmed because the doctor said I had fibroids – but he said there was absolutely nothing to worry about.'

On the other hand, symptoms may sometimes be ignored by doctors or put down to other conditions.

Joan's story

Joan's fibroid symptoms were initially misdiagnosed ten years ago, when she was in her early twenties. 'I went into hospital because I was in great pain. I was in and out of there for a week before they made the correct diagnosis. At first I was given drugs for a urinary tract infection, then drugs for a kidney infection. They then decided that I needed to have my appendix out. Luckily the operation couldn't be done immediately because I had eaten some food. A gynaecologist then examined me, looked at my case-notes and said that the diagnosis was wrong. He explained that I had fibroids.'

Janet's story

Forty-one-year-old Janet started getting low back pains and abdominal cramps after the birth of her son, five years ago. 'I had been fine up till the pregnancy, but afterwards I developed these symptoms which I put down to pregnancy and childbirth. The problems persisted, and I also started getting rather lumpy round my middle. I went to see my GP who decided I was depressed and put me on an antidepressant. Eventually I insisted on seeing a

31

gynaecologist. On examining me, he said I had fibroids and that my womb was the size of a 16-week pregnancy.'

Jill's story

Jill, 50, had a similar experience in her early twenties, when she was having heavy periods. She became very anaemic and was tearful a lot of the time. 'I went to see my GP who told me to put up with the heavy bleeding. He gave me antidepressants. I thought something else must be wrong, and I went to see my doctor again. Fortunately he wasn't there and I saw another doctor, who agreed to refer me to a specialist who diagnosed fibroids.'

Rachel's story

Rachel, aged 40, had heavy periods in her late twenties. 'I thought this was normal. However, at one point I went to my GP about the problem. I saw a locum doctor who didn't examine me, but just advised me to go on the Pill. I didn't want to do this, so I put up with the problem. I went back and saw my own GP some time later to have a general check-up, because I wanted to get pregnant. I mentioned that I had heavy periods, and my GP did an internal examination. He told me I had fibroids, but that I would need further tests to confirm the diagnosis.'

If you have symptoms, it is important to get a check-up. It's unlikely to be anything serious. You may have fibroids – or, very occasionally, the symptoms could be a sign of something more serious. As we have seen, ovarian cancer occurs most often in post-menopausal women, though it can occur in younger women. It causes vague symptoms, one of which may be a swollen abdomen. The earlier the cancer is treated, the better the outlook.

Go to see your GP and discuss your symptoms. Your doctor is likely to do an initial examination and then refer you to a gynaecologist, a doctor who specializes in the female reproductive system. If you are unhappy with the gynaecologist's diagnosis, talk to your GP about getting a second opinion from another gynaecologist. Issues about how to get the best help are discussed in more detail in Chapter 5.

It is important to get a proper diagnosis. In the past, more mistakes were made because diagnostic techniques were not so good. Today, diagnosis is more accurate because of improved diagnostic tests. Many of the procedures you are likely to have are simple and safe – though some do have a small risk attached to them. Those procedures which penetrate the body in any way are called invasive, and always include a slight risk of infection or damage to surrounding body-tissue. If you are worried about anything to do with the tests, talk about your anxieties to your GP or the specialist who is treating you. Find out if the test is really necessary, and what it will reveal. Ask how accurate the test is, what risks (if any) are attached to it, and if there are better and safer tests available.

When you get the diagnosis, try to find out as much as you can about where the fibroids are located, how many there are and their size. Most women I spoke to just knew they had fibroids, but nothing more. But this information is important in order to help you understand why you are getting symptoms, as well as in helping you to discuss treatment options with your doctor.

Tests

Your GP will want to know about your symptoms. Before you go along, it's worth noting down specific details about your problems. For example, if your symptom is heavy and painful periods, note what you mean by this. For instance, have they always been heavy? Has there been some change in blood-flow? Does bleeding last longer? What sort of pain do you have, and when does it start and finish? Have you started passing clots?

Clinical examination

Every woman I spoke to had this examination, and for some it was the only diagnostic test. This is the usual way of starting investigations, and can often reveal whether there are fibroids. Further tests are then sometimes done to confirm the diagnosis, and to give more information about the fibroids.

You will be asked to remove clothes below the waist and lie down on the examination table with your knees bent. First, the doctor will gently press your abdominal wall. If the fibroid is quite large, the doctor may be able to feel the lump – but not know exactly where it is in the pelvis.

The doctor will go on to do an internal examination to try and get more detailed information about what is happening inside your pelvis.

Many women feel understandably anxious about this intimate procedure. The examination shouldn't hurt – but if you are tense, relax by breathing through your abdomen (a technique discussed in more detail in Chapter 10). If you feel any pain, tell the doctor immediately. If you have a pelvic infection you may, for example, feel very tender.

The internal examination is called bimanual because it is done with two hands (see Figure 2). One hand rests on your abdomen, just above the pubic bone, while one or two lubricated fingers of the other hand are gently inserted into the vagina. By pushing upwards on the cervix and pressing down gently on the abdomen, the doctor can check the size and position of the womb and the ovaries, and can detect any abnormal pelvic swelling or tenderness. Large fibroids can often be detected this way. The doctor will also be checking the tissue either side of the womb, known as the adnexa. If a lump is discovered in this area, it's called an adnexal mass. The doctor then has to decide whether it is an ovarian or tubal lump, or a fibroid in the broad ligament. If the doctor is confident that you have fibroids, and if they are not causing you any problems, then no further tests may be needed. But you may be referred for an ultrasound scan if there is any uncertainty about the diagnosis or if more information is needed about the fibroids in order to make treatment decisions.

Ultrasound scan

Before the invention of ultrasound scanning, diagnosis was based on the internal examination – and more operations were carried out just to check what was going on inside the abdomen. The internal examination cannot easily distinguish between ovarian problems and an enlarged womb with fibroids.

Judy's story

Judy, 44, had a internal examination and ultrasound scanning a year ago. 'I didn't have any fibroid symptoms, but I had a cervical smear done last year and the nurse referred me to the GP because my womb felt a bit bulky. The doctor did an internal examination and said, 'There's something there' – and referred me to a gynaecologist. I had another internal, and also an abdominal ultrasound scan which confirmed I had a fibroid the size of a grapefruit.'

34

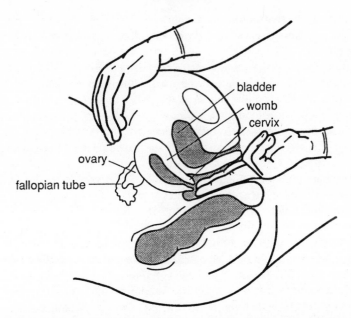

bladder
womb
cervix
ovary
fallopian tube

Figure 2 A routine bimanual (two-handed) pelvic examination can detect a womb which is enlarged or distorted by fibroids.

Nowadays, an abdominal ultrasound scan is the most widely used procedure for investigating pelvic masses (the term used by doctor for lumps in that part of the body). The scan is generally accurate, and gives a detailed picture of the size and position of fibroids in the womb. Results are good when it's done by a specialist experienced in gynaecological ultrasound. In four large studies, ultrasound was able correctly to diagnose fibroids in 88 per cent of cases. The scan should also be able to detect whether there is any fluid in the abdomen, which could suggest ovarian problems. It can also show whether there is any pressure on the ureters. If the scan shows this, you will need intravenous urography (discussed later in this chapter) to find out whether the fibroid or something like a stone is causing the obstruction.

Abdominal ultrasound is good at giving information about large fibroids, but less good at detecting small fibroids. However, a vaginal ultrasound scan can do this, so doctors may use a combination of abdominal and vaginal ultrasound scans to assess your fibroids. Some radiologists (doctors who are trained in using imaging techniques like

35

ultrasound) say that vaginal ultrasound scans can detect most fibroids, and that abdominal scans are only needed if there is a large mass in the abdomen.

Ultrasound uses very high-frequency sound-waves, which are passed into the body. Echoes from the sound-waves are built into a picture of the inside of the abdomen, which can be seen on a television screen. It's possible to build up a three-dimensional 'map' of what the fibroids are like and where they are located. Fibroids have specific characteristics which enable them to be distinguished from other pelvic conditions, such as ovarian cysts.

An abdominal ultrasound scan is painless. But you do need a full bladder, which can be a nuisance, and you will be told to drink up to a litre of fluid before your appointment. If you have to wait for your appointment, you may feel rather uncomfortable – and it's possible that, when you get to see the doctor, you may still be told your bladder isn't full enough. You may have to drink more and have a further wait until your bladder is full. A probe covered in gel is then moved over your abdomen to produce the picture. Abdominal ultrasound is a good detection test provided you're not too fat – which can make it less accurate.

Vaginal ultrasound can get closer to the fibroids, and so gives better detail about the growths. A probe measuring a few centimetres across is put into your vagina. It may be a bit uncomfortable when the probe is pushed against the top of vagina to get a better picture of the ovaries. But the procedure is painless and no sedative is needed. You don't need a full bladder for this procedure.

Other tests

A simple blood-test is usually done to check for anaemia. A sample is taken from a vein in your arm to look at haemoglobin-levels in your blood. The doctor may also ask the laboratory to check on blood ferritin levels, to assess the amount of iron stored in your body. Ask your doctor if you can have these tests done, as many women are anaemic without knowing it.

The doctor may also get a blood-test done to look at certain hormone-levels, to find out how near you are to the menopause – as this may affect treatment decisions. The menopause (which is when you stop having periods) technically means your last period. It usually happens at some point from your late forties to mid-fifties. Before it occurs, hormone-levels start to change over a number of years. Levels of oestrogen start to fall from the mid-thirties onwards. The pituitary gland starts to produce higher levels of FSH (follicle-stimulating hormone), in order to try and stimulate the ovaries into egg production. Low oestrogen-levels and high FSH-levels indicate that your body is preparing for the menopause. However, the information can't predict how long this phase will last.

Tests may also be done to check how well your thyroid is functioning. The thyroid is an important gland which produces hormones that regulate energy levels. An underactive thyroid can also cause heavy bleeding.

A range of other tests will be done if you have bladder or bowel symptoms, to find out what's causing the problem. Your urine may be analysed, and checks may be done for blood in bowel movements. Intravenous urography, also known as intravenous pyelography, is a procedure for obtaining X-rays of the urinary tract, which is made up of the bladder, kidneys and ureters. You will be told not to drink for four hours beforehand, and given a laxative to empty the bowels. A special substance which shows up on an X-ray is injected through a vein in your arm. Timed X-rays are taken after the injection, to show up possible blockages in the urinary tract as the substance starts to move through it.

Magnetic Resonance Imaging

It's unlikely that you will have an MRI (Magnetic Resonance Imaging) scan, as the other tests normally give an accurate diagnosis. Also, though MRI is more accurate than ultrasound, it is very expensive and the machines are in short supply. But MRI can be done if, after the ultrasound scan, there is still uncertainty about what is going on inside the pelvis. For example, it can sometimes be difficult to distinguish an ovarian cyst pressed against the womb from a fibroid. MRI can differentiate between the two, as well as distinguishing between normal and abnormal tissue. It can also distinguish between fibroids and adenomyosis.

MRI is a diagnostic technique which provides three-dimensional images of organs and structures inside the body without using X-rays or other radiation. The scan carries no known side-effects or risks because it doesn't use radiation.

To have an MRI test, you lie inside a huge, hollow cylindrical magnet, surrounded by a large electromagnet, and are exposed to bursts of powerful magnetic fields and radio-waves. These stimulate your body to emit radio signals which are detected and analysed by a computer to create an image of a section of your body. The scan may take about 30 minutes to do, and you need to lie very still. MRI is usually done on an outpatient basis. No metal objects are allowed inside the room, so you'll be asked to remove items such as watches, hairgrips and jewellery. If you feel worried about being isolated inside the tube, tell the person who is doing the test. They can see and hear you all the time.

Transvaginal guided biopsy

Radiologists work on the principle that fibroids are non-cancerous. But very occasionally, a fibroid may have suspicious signs: it may be growing fast or, instead of having the usual whorled appearance of benign growths, it may look like raw pork.

As discussed in Chapter 3, your gynaecologist will want to do a hysterectomy if the fibroid is clearly cancerous. But if there is a question-mark, the doctor will want a biopsy – that is, a tissue sample – so that it can be checked in the laboratory. An operation is done to remove the whole fibroid, and if it is cancerous, a second operation will be done to remove the womb.

But a few centres are using a less invasive technique, known as transvaginal guided biopsy, to collect the tissue sample. The technique is slightly painful, so you may be given a sedative which will be injected into a vein in your hand or arm. A needle is fired from a special instrument, about a centimetre wide, through the wall at the top of the vagina next to the neck of the womb; it collects the sample from the centre of the fibroid. The procedure takes about 15 minutes. You may have a bit of spotting or pass clots for a day or two afterwards. Results take a couple of days to come through.

The disadvantage of this, as one specialist explained, is that cancerous changes might not spread evenly throughout the fibroid. He was concerned that a fibroid could be cancerous even though the tissue sample was normal. Where malignancy is suspected, he would therefore always want the whole fibroid removed and checked for signs of cancer. Some doctors may also want to proceed straightaway to hysterectomy, rather than doing a biopsy, if there's any possibility of cancer. Issues about treatment choice are discussed in Chapter 5.

Cervical smear

Various checks will be done for abnormal bleeding or irregular spotting, to rule out the possibility of other cancers. A cervical smear will probably be taken, depending on when you last had one done, to check that the cervix is healthy.

D&C

There are now several ways of checking the womb-lining for abnormalities. Whether or not your doctor wants to do this depends on your symptoms and age. But if you're under 40, you are very unlikely to have cancer of the womb-lining.

In the past a D&C (dilatation and curettage) would have been done to check for cancer of the womb-lining. A D&C is a blind scrape of the womb-lining, usually done under general anaesthetic (though it can be done under local anaesthetic). The neck of the womb is opened gradually and a spoon-shaped instrument called a curette is passed into the womb. The lining is scraped away and sent off for examination.

Afterwards you may have some bleeding for several days, and mild pain. If you have got fibroids, the bleeding may be heavier. Don't use tampons to reduce the risk of infection – and watch out for signs of infection, which include cramping pains, a smelly discharge and increased bleeding. It's important not to make love until the bleeding and discharge have gone. Your periods may take a couple of months or so to get back to normal.

D&Cs used to be routinely used as a diagnostic procedure on many women. They were also thought to be a useful treatment, because it was claimed problems often got better when D&Cs were done. About 140,000 D&Cs are performed each year, but D&Cs have come in for criticism in the last few years. Researchers now say it is an ineffective technique which should not be used in women under 40, because womb-cancer is so unlikely in younger women. Some researchers argue that it is a crude diagnostic tool, and that problems may be missed because the surgeon does a blind scrape. There's also little evidence that it works as a treatment.

Endometrial sample

Newer ways of taking samples are simpler, less invasive and as accurate, according to some research. A tiny sampling device is inserted into the womb through the cervix, and tissue is gently extracted and taken away for inspection. A general anaesthetic is not needed, and the sample can be taken on an outpatient basis. It's similar to having a cervical smear done. You lie on your back, knees bent, legs apart and let your knees flop down on either side. An instrument called a speculum, which opens up the vagina, is inserted. A tiny, hollow tube with a plunger is then inserted through the neck of the womb, which doesn't have to be widened, into the womb-cavity. Using the device, the doctor cuts off a tiny piece of womb-lining and draws it into the tube. The procedure shouldn't be painful, though you may feel some period-like cramps when the sample is being taken.

Hysteroscopy

The best way to check the womb-lining is by looking at it, according to many gynaecologists. Some doctors now do this routinely if there are any suspicious symptoms. A hysteroscope is a fine viewing-instrument, slightly thicker than a ball-point pen (about a centimetre wide), which can be used to look at the inside of the womb. It's passed through the vagina and up into the womb through the neck of the womb, which has to be gently widened. The hysteroscope has various channels in it: one through which the doctor inspects the inside of the womb; another to insert gas and fluid which separate the womb-walls to give a good view inside; and others through which instruments are passed, to take a biopsy of any suspicious-looking tissue. Hysteroscopy is done on an outpatient basis, and you should be able to go home afterwards.

Some women find the procedure relatively painless – but you may experience some pain. Women who have had children may not find the procedure so painful. A local anaesthetic is injected into the neck of the womb, or a light general anaesthetic may be used.

Susan's story

Susan, 44, had a hysteroscopy a couple of years ago. 'It took about 20 minutes but was incredibly painful, even though I'd had a local anaesthetic. I had to be given more pain relief. Afterwards I was fine.'

The advantage of the procedure is that the gynaecologist can see what's inside, and remove specific tissue for analysis. The doctor can usually see whether there are any fibroids – although this is not always the case. Susan's womb was so distorted that the fibroids could not be seen.

The doctor may also discover polyps. These are non-cancerous growths in the neck of the womb or the womb-lining, which, like fibroids, can cause irregular bleeding and bleeding after love-making, as well as heavy periods – but not the other fibroid symptoms. One study found that ultrasound was unable to distinguish between fibroids and polyps, so the doctor may want to do a hysteroscopy. Fibroids and polyps can be removed using a hysteroscope (this is discussed in Chapter 7).

Hysterosalpingogram

Some gynaecologists use this procedure – known as HSG for short – for women with known or suspected fibroids who want to get pregnant, or who have a history of losing pregnancies. It can check the inside of the womb and also show whether there are blockages inside the Fallopian tubes. In the past, HSG was the gold standard for identifying submucous fibroids. Nowadays there are alternatives, such as hysteroscopy (as just discussed), which allows the doctor to look inside the womb and also take samples if necessary; there is also laparoscopy (discussed below), which allows the doctor to look directly into the abdomen, at the outside of the Fallopian tubes and womb.

HSG is an X-ray procedure which is usually done on an outpatient basis. A teaspoonful of a special dye which shows up on X-ray, is injected slowly into the womb through a tiny tube inserted into the cervix. This can be unpleasant, but if the dye is injected very slowly – which takes about 30 minutes – there shouldn't be any pain, according to an eminent infertility specialist. He comments that about one in four women experience momentary discomfort, which should pass after about ten minutes. According to him, the pain should never be unbearable.

Laura's story

Laura has had two HSGs. 'I was frightened the first time because I didn't know what to expect. But I was fine. I had some pain afterwards, for about eight hours which I treated with paracetamol. Two years later I had another HSG. This was an awful experience. My womb was so large by then that they had had to keep putting more and more dye into me, and this is what made it so painful I think.'

You may need a day or so to get back to normal. Also, expect a dye-coloured discharge – so use sanitary pads. Tell the doctor if you have a history of allergies (such as asthma and hay fever), as occasionally it is possible to have an allergic response to the dye. An old infection may start up again after an HSG, so tell your doctor if you have had a recent pelvic infection; bad vaginal discharge; tenderness on pelvic examination; increasing pain when making love. If this is the case, you may be given a course of antibiotics and the procedure postponed.

Laparoscopy

Laparoscopy is a good way of checking what is going on inside the abdomen. It's usually carried out under general anaesthetic, though it can be done under a local. Used as a diagnostic test, it can look at the outside of the womb and the Fallopian tubes, and take samples of tissue for analysis if necessary. It can be used to confirm a diagnosis and to check for conditions such as endometriosis. It is also used to do operations (this is discussed in Chapter 7).

The advantage of a laparoscopy is that the abdomen is punctured rather than cut open. This makes recovery very quick. A tiny, centimetre-wide puncture is made underneath the navel, and harmless carbon dioxide gas is pumped into the abdomen through a hollow tube, to inflate the cavity. This makes it easier to see the womb and ovaries inside the pelvis. The laparoscope, another type of viewing-instrument, is then inserted through another tiny puncture. If other instruments are used, these are inserted through one or two other tiny incisions above the pubic bone. A probe is also inserted into your womb through the neck of the womb. The probe is used to move the womb slightly backwards and forwards, so that the surgeon can see it from various angles.

The procedure should take about 30 minutes, and you will have one or two stitches afterwards. These may dissolve on their own or may need to be removed by the surgeon or your doctor a few days later. After a couple of hours you should be able to go home. The gas may make you feel bloated and a bit uncomfortable for a day or two, and you may also have some discomfort in the chest and some pain around the shoulder due to the gas. This is called *referred pain*, because the gas tends to irritate the nerves supplying the abdomen and chest-wall. A simple painkiller should help ease the discomfort.

Like any invasive procedure, laparoscopy has risks. The womb, bladder or bowel are damaged very occasionally, and there is a risk of infection developing. Tell your doctor if you develop any of the following: constant pain, fever, vomiting, heavy and persistent vaginal bleeding, bad-smelling vaginal discharge, problems passing urine or opening your bowels.

The surgeon may also not be able to see much if there is a lot of scar-tissue inside your abdomen – perhaps from previous surgery, or an infection, or if you are very overweight. In this case, the surgeon may end up doing a conventional operation called a laparotomy (discussed in more detail in Chapter 7), in order to see inside the abdomen properly. But the surgeon should warn you beforehand about this possibility, which may be more likely if you have had previous pelvic surgery. Talk to the surgeon to find out your chances of this happening.

Summary

Nowadays, various diagnostic techniques, which are relatively non-invasive, can be used to find out what is going on inside your abdomen. The tests can confirm or disprove a provisional diagnosis of fibroids, and can give more information about the lumps. Other pelvic conditions – such as ovarian cysts and endometriosis – can be detected. No diagnostic test is perfect, and it may be important to have a mix of tests in order to get a proper diagnosis. Diagnostic tests also carry risks, and it's possible that occasionally a laparoscopy could end up turning into a bigger operation.

5

Treatment – general issues

What should you do if fibroids are diagnosed? In the past, before the introduction of the various diagnostic techniques just discussed, doctors often tended to recommend surgery because they were worried about the possibility of cancer in the pelvic area. But with today's diagnostic techniques, the doctor can usually get a good idea of what is going on inside the pelvis without having to resort to major surgery.

There is no need to rush into any treatment suggested, and it's important to take time and think through what you want, in consultation with your doctor. But your gynaecologist will want to operate as soon as possible if there is cancer anywhere in the pelvis.

Relationship with doctors

Nowadays there are more options about what treatment to have. It's important to recognize that doctors will have different views about the various treatments, depending on their experience, interests and expertise. Some will have kept up-to-date with the latest techniques, but others may offer outdated advice – for example, that a hysterectomy is always necessary.

Lucy's story

Lucy's fibroids were discovered when she was 36. 'I was living abroad at the time, and the gynaecologist did an internal examination and said I had fibroids. He was very worried about them, and told me I might need a blood transfusion and that I should come home as soon as possible as I would need to have a hysterectomy. I was very worried, so I came back to the UK and saw another gynaecologist who confirmed the original diagnosis. But he wasn't at all alarmed by the fibroids and didn't prescribe any treatment.'

Treatment choices

Everyone is different, and some women may not want to discuss treatment options, preferring just to go ahead with whatever their doctor suggests. But many women increasingly want to be involved in decisions which could significantly affect their lives. If you feel like this, make time to talk through treatment options with the doctors responsible for your care. Doctors, for their part, are increasingly keen to do this as they recognize that patients often get upset because of communication difficulties between doctor and patient.

Some doctors are very good at discussing treatment options, and others are less so. Treatments all have advantages and disadvantages. Doctors will also have different views about what should be done.

Rachel's story

Rachel says: 'I saw a very good consultant after I'd found out that fibroids were causing my heavy bleeding. She gave me several options: I could do nothing, or I could think about having an operation to remove the fibroids because I wanted to have children. She mentioned a hysterectomy, but said this was the last option and would probably be unnecessary in my case.'

Sarah's story

Sarah, 52, was unhappy about the advice she was given last year. 'I went to see a female gynaecologist who told me I had a huge fibroid the size of a melon and that I would need a hysterectomy straightaway. She started flicking through her diary for a date. I was stunned and told her I was going to be away on holiday shortly. She said she wouldn't advise this, and told me that I was very anaemic, implying that I would die unless I had an immediate blood transfusion. She offered me no alternative options. She made out that a hysterectomy was an easy procedure and that I would only need six weeks off work. But I didn't want to have another major operation unless I absolutely needed one. I had recently had time off work for an eye operation. I also hoped that, because of my age, I might be able to make it to the menopause without having surgery. The gynaecologist also wanted to take my ovaries out during the hysterectomy, but I didn't want this done because I thought this might give me acute menopausal symptoms.

'I was very upset after the appointment. I felt as though she was bulldozing me into having the operation. I had the blood transfusion and then saw my GP, who arranged for me to see another consultant for a second opinion. This doctor was very different in his approach. He took time discussing drug and surgical options with me, and though we didn't agree on everything, I didn't feel upset. He thought it was a good idea for me to think things over and said that it made sense for me to have a holiday as I needed time to recover after losing all that blood.'

Angela's story

Angela was very pleased when her fibroid was removed. 'But I was never told that there might be different ways of removing it, or that it might regrow after surgery. I was also not given any information about drug treatments as a possible alternative to surgery.'

Talk to your GP about treatment choices. If you feel ill-at-ease with your own doctor and belong to a group practice, try to see one of the other doctors – but if you can't find a sympathetic GP in the practice, you could think about changing to another practice. In theory you have the right to do so easily and quickly, according to the Patient's Charter, but in reality this may not be so easy.

You are also not obliged to have any treatment recommended by your doctor. The Patient's Charter gives you the right to have any proposed treatment explained to you, with details of its risks and of possible alternative treatments. You can stop treatment at any time, even if you have signed a consent form. If you are worried about any of these issues and want more information, talk to your local community health council or Healthpoint, an NHS telephone advice service (details are at the back of the book). But it's very likely that you will be able to sort out any worries with your doctor.

Nowadays doctors do take more note of what women want. In the past, many took the view that women who had completed their families or were nearing the menopause would be happy to have a hysterectomy. But doctors did recognize that women wanting children would not want to have their womb removed unless absolutely necessary. So an operation called a myomectomy was developed, which removes only the fibroids.

What you want will depend on various things – such as your age, what sort of symptoms you have, their severity and how long you have had them, your past experience of surgery, your feelings about having a major operation and how you view your body. Doctors can sometimes find it hard to grasp that some women do not want to have their womb out, even if they have completed their family or are never going to have children. These women may not like the idea of losing what they see as an essential part of themselves. For them, a hysterectomy is not the obvious solution. Yet others are only too happy to have a hysterectomy. Some of these views are reflected in more detail in Chapter 8.

Finding a gynaecologist

Your GP is very likely to refer you to a gynaecologist for confirmation of the diagnosis and for discussion of treatment options, if appropriate. It's possible that your GP may treat you initially. But a gynaecologist gets involved for more specialist drug treatment, or if surgery is needed.

What happens if your GP is not prepared to refer you to a specialist? Under the Patient's Charter you have a right to be referred to a consultant, but only when your GP thinks this is necessary. So you don't have an absolute right, according to the Charter. The simplest way round this is to see another GP if you are in a group practice. Another route might be to consider going to a Well Woman clinic. (Again, ring Healthpoint and other groups listed at the back of the book for more information.) However, most GPs will want to refer you to a gynaecologist so that your symptoms can be thoroughly investigated.

Choosing a gynaecologist

How can you ensure that you see a gynaecologist who is experienced in the treatment of fibroids? This is a difficult question with no easy answers. Your GP will know the local gynaecologists, and will suggest one – it's worth asking, at the outset, to see one with a special interest in fibroids. If you see a gynaecologist who is not experienced in this area, ask to be referred to a colleague who is experienced in treating fibroids. If this doesn't happen, talk to your GP about seeing another gynaecologist. Some hospitals also have specialist clinics for heavy bleeding, and you may be referred to one of these. This issue becomes more important if you have particularly problematic fibroids or want to find out about the latest treatment approaches.

There are other ways of finding gynaecologists who have special expertise in the area. You may find it useful to look at *The Good Doctor Guide* by Catherine Vassallo. This lists the qualifications and interests of various types of specialists in the country.

Articles in magazines and newspapers on fibroids may include quotes from consultants with a particular interest in the subject. Medical journals – such as the *British Medical Journal*, *The Lancet* and the *British Journal of Obstetrics and Gynaecology* – are worth looking at: gynaecologists with a special interest in fibroids sometimes write articles in these journals from time to time. Medical-school libraries hold these journals, so you could try ringing the librarian and asking whether you could come along to look at them. If you identify a specialist, you could contact their secretary and ask how you go about seeing the specialist.

You may want to see a consultant who works in another Health Authority area. But your Authority would have to agree to pay for this under a system known as extra-contractual referral payments. However, some authorities are cutting back on these payments. If your Health Authority refuses to make a special payment, get advice from your local community health council. But be warned: there are no easy solutions. If you belong to a fundholding GP practice, your doctor may pay for you to see a gynaecologist elsewhere.

Louise's story

Louise, aged 41, had a recurrence of fibroid symptoms a year ago. She was having bad period-cramps and non-stop flooding, and saw a specialist who removed her fibroids using the latest surgical techniques. 'I went privately so I did have more choice – but I still made sure I found the best possible doctor to do the operation. The same point applies if you're getting NHS treatment, though it may be harder to do what I did. You need to check the surgeon out beforehand, just like you would a car mechanic. I decided to ring the local hospitals and spoke to the administrators for information about gynaecologists and their skills. One person's name kept coming up. He was apparently very experienced in fibroid surgery, so I decided to see him before having the operation – though I think it's unusual to do this, and some doctors may not like this approach.

I asked him various questions and decided I could trust him. He agreed to operate and everything went very well.'

If the gynaecologist advises you to have a particular surgical treatment, ask what experience they have of performing the procedure. This is particularly important with the latest keyhole surgical techniques, which involve making tiny cuts rather than big incisions in the abdomen. These procedures have advantages because they appear less invasive, and recovery time is quicker – but they can be very risky in untrained hands. The Royal College of Obstetricians and Gynaecologists is developing a system whereby surgeons are awarded certificates of competence in the various techniques.

Take time to think things over, and remember you can't be forced to have treatment. If you're unhappy with the consultant you see, you have the right to a second opinion – but again, only if your GP thinks this is desirable.

Consent to surgery

The hospital will give you a consent form to sign, which in effect allows the surgeon to do whatever they think necessary at the time of the operation. If you are having a hysterectomy, the doctor may talk to you about removing your ovaries. These may have to be taken out if they are diseased. But some doctors think it's best to take out healthy ovaries in women nearing the menopause, because of the danger of ovarian cancer developing later on. (This is discussed in more detail in Chapter 8).

Some women are happy about this – but you may not want this done for reasons which are discussed in Chapter 8. In practice, there is no fail-safe way of preventing the surgeon removing your ovaries. The doctor can always argue that it was necessary to do this during the operation because of unforeseen complications which put you at risk, and that it was done with the best of intentions. When you sign the consent form, you could add a note saying that under no circumstances are your ovaries to be removed. You could also cross out the section which allows the surgeon the right to decide what should be done during surgery. However the surgeon is then very unlikely to want to perform the operation.

The best way of dealing with your concerns, and minimizing the chances of your ovaries being removed is to talk to the surgeon who is going to do the operation. But it isn't always easy to know who is going to operate – it may not be the gynaecologist who deals with you. All being well, the surgeon will also want to speak to you beforehand, so you should have a chance to discuss your worries. Finally, if you think your wishes may not be respected, you could always decide not to have the operation.

Treatment options

How good is the treatment?

The effectiveness of treatment is a vital issue. Researchers funded by the NHS are looking increasingly at the effectiveness of all kinds of treatments – the NHS does not want to pay for costly treatments which may be ineffective. As many as four out of five treatments have not been properly evaluated to find out whether or not they work. Doctors often prescribe treatments out of habit, personal experience and medical-school training which could be out of date.

Research into gynaecological treatments so far suggests that, as already mentioned, diagnostic D&C should not be carried out on women under 40. Evidence also shows that the drugs most often prescribed for heavy periods by GPs are the least effective ones. About five per cent of women aged 30 – 49 consult their GP about the problem, and about 822,000 prescriptions were handed out in 1993. For heavy bleeding, GPs often prescribe low doses of a drug called norethisterone – but one research study found that this could actually increase bleeding by 20 per cent.

So ask about the benefits, risks and side-effects of any treatment your doctor suggests to you. Also ask about alternative treatments.

HRT

If you have troublesome fibroids, and want HRT to help with menopausal symptoms, your doctor may be reluctant to prescribe it in case it makes the fibroids grow. A doctor may recommend a hysterectomy so that HRT can be safely used – a difficult choice for a woman who doesn't want surgery and isn't seeking fibroid treatment, but merely wants help with the menopause.

Lucy's story

Despite her fibroid symptoms, Lucy was hoping to make it to the menopause without having to have surgery. 'I went to my gynaecologist to talk about having HRT and was very surprised when he said I would need a hysterectomy if I wanted HRT. He said my womb was the size of a 16-week pregnancy, and that HRT would make it even bigger. I've reluctantly decided to have the operation because I want to take HRT for my menopausal symptoms. I've also got some fibroid symptoms so maybe the operation makes sense.'

HRT gives you oestradiol – the type of oestrogen which is lost once the ovaries stop producing oestrogen after the menopause. In post-menopausal women, oestradiol-levels decrease to around 10 per cent of previous levels – though the other types of oestrogen remain at a fairly steady level. After the menopause, oestrogens come from fat-cells which convert adrenal hormones (particularly androstenedione) to oestrogen. Fatter post-menopausal women thus have higher oestrogen-levels than thinner women.

As hormone-levels change around the menopause, women can suffer distressing symptoms – such as hot flushes, night sweats, vaginal and bladder problems. In the long term, as a result of having lower amounts of the powerful type of oestrogen, women can become more susceptible to the bone-thinning disease osteoporosis, and to heart disease.

HRT replaces the oestrogen which post-menopausal women have lost. If a woman still has her womb, she is given HRT which also contains progestogen, to make sure that cancer of the womb-lining does not develop. HRT contains lower doses of oestrogen than the contraceptive Pill, and can be taken in various ways. It can relieve short-term symptoms and protect against longer-term problems. But there is a debate about the side-effects and risks of HRT treatment: some women cannot take it and some women do not want to take it. Alternatives to HRT are discussed in Chapter 10.

Specialists have different views about whether you should take HRT if you have had symptomatic fibroids (that is, fibroids which give rise to symptoms – as opposed to unsymptomatic fibroids, which cause no problems). Some say that the oestrogen in HRT increases fibroid size and brings back troublesome symptoms. However, this did not happen in a study (reported in the journal *Fertility and Sterility*, February 1996), in which researchers looked at two groups of women taking different types of HRT. They noted that the fibroids did increase in size in one group – but that none of the women were troubled by any symptoms.

I spoke to several doctors to try and clarify whether HRT can make fibroids more troublesome. One specialist pointed out that HRT preparations vary a lot, and are taken in different ways. The implication was that some types of HRT might possibly promote fibroid growth, whereas others might not – and that more research is needed to find out which HRT preparations might be more problematic. The following points emerged from my discussions with two doctors with a special interest in the subject.

- It's not necessary to have a hysterectomy if you have symptomatic fibroids and want to take HRT. HRT is fine for 95 per cent of women in this category.

- It's difficult to know which women are going to have difficulties as a result of taking HRT – but it's likely to be those who have had large, problematic fibroids for some years. However this doesn't always happen. I was told of one case where a woman had a troublesome, large fibroid but was very keen to take HRT. The doctor reluctantly prescribed HRT, fearing that she might experience heavy periods. But the woman has had no bleeding problems and has now been on HRT for several years.

- Doctors worry that HRT withdrawal bleeds may become heavier – but some women can now side-step withdrawal bleeds. HRT is made up of oestrogen and progestogen taken as separate pills. Oestrogen increases the womb-lining in a process which, if unchecked, could lead to cancer of the womb-lining. So progestogen is given, usually for about 12 days each month, so that the lining is shed as a period. But there is no withdrawal bleed if a form of HRT is taken which combines both hormones together in one pill. The lining doesn't build up, so there is no risk of cancer and no womb-lining to shed. The drug is restricted to women over 50, or those whose last period was at least a year previously.

- Fibroids which have not caused problems in the past should not become troublesome when you take HRT.

- Troublesome fibroids are unlikely to grow unless you are very unlucky – though they may shrink more slowly with HRT.
- If you do take HRT, fibroids can be monitored with ultrasound to check what is happening to them.
- The aim should be to take the lowest possible dose of oestrogen so that it relieves menopausal symptoms but doesn't encourage fibroid growth.

Symptoms and treatments: some points to consider

- If the fibroids are causing no problems, treatment is unnecessary. Some doctors don't think it's necessary to keep an eye on fibroids; others may want to monitor the fibroids with ultrasound on a regular basis. You may find this reassuring – but not everyone wants this.

Helen's story

Helen, in her mid-thirties, who has twice had operations to remove her fibroids, says: 'I know they have regrown and are there, but I'm fine at the moment. I've got the two children I wanted. There's no point monitoring the fibroids. I'm too busy. If they start to become a nuisance, I'll sort the problems out then.'

- If you want children and have fibroids, it is important to talk to an infertility specialist about whether the fibroids could be affecting your fertility.
- Fibroids in pregnancy are not generally a major problem and are often detected when you have a routine scan. It's not usually necessary to remove fibroids if you're planning to get pregnant.
- In the unlikely event that your doctor recommends surgery on the basis that fibroids can become cancerous, remember that this is very rare and is more likely in women past the menopause. The warning signs, as discussed in Chapter 3, include a sudden growth-spurt (though this is not always a sign of a malignant fibroid). If you have worrying symptoms, and if imaging techniques suggest that the fibroid is abnormal, then a tissue sample will be needed. Most doctors say it's best to remove the whole fibroid rather than a small part of it, in order to judge whether the fibroid is cancerous.
- If you have got symptoms it's worth thinking about several points. Is your doctor certain that the fibroids are responsible for the

symptoms? It may be that some other gynaecological condition is causing the problem. It's always important, therefore, to get a proper diagnosis as outlined in the last chapter. In the past, doctors tried to remove all fibroids, regardless of whether they were causing problems. Some doctors now just remove the fibroids they think are causing problems and leave the others behind.

- Whether or not you decide on treatment will depend on what the problem is, how long you have had it and whether you feel you can cope with it. This is obviously a personal decision. Some women, for example, would prefer to cope with heavy periods, whereas others may want to have a hysterectomy.

Mary's story

Fifty-year-old Mary wants a hysterectomy. 'I've had lots of difficulties with my fibroids since I was in my mid-twenties. I had one operation to remove them. My health improved afterwards for a time, but my periods started to get heavier again and I began having uncontrollable bleeding for the first three days of my period. Tests showed that the fibroids had regrown. They've been monitored with ultrasound over the years and I've also had a D&C to try and help the bleeding-problems. A couple of years ago I asked about the possibility of having everything taken out, but I was told my problems weren't severe enough to justify a hysterectomy.'

- Nowadays there are a range of treatment options, so discuss these with your doctor. You may just need drugs which provide symptom relief.
- Symptoms can vary over time. If you develop fibroids at a young age, there is more time for them to become troublesome before the menopause. But they don't inevitably get worse, and there may be ups and downs in the severity of symptoms.

Sarah's story

Sarah's heavy periods started when she was about 37 and were very heavy for about three years. 'Then everything got better until I was in my late forties, but unfortunately the bleeding slowly started getting worse again.'

- If you're coming up to the menopause you may find that you can manage to cope, with the help of drug treatment, until you stop having periods. There are drugs which can shrink fibroids and relieve symptoms, but they are expensive and have side-effects. (They are discussed in Chapter 6). However, as already mentioned, it's difficult to know how long the run-up to the menopause will last.

Summary

- Ask about the risks and side-effects of any proposed treatment. Check if there are any alternative treatments and ask how they compare with one another. Find out what the success rates are for the various treatments. If surgery is advised, try to find out how experienced the surgeon is at carrying out that particular procedure.
- Try to speak to the person carrying out surgery so that you can discuss any wishes or worries you may have.
- Give yourself time to think about treatment options.
- HRT can normally be taken if you have fibroids, and the fibroids can be monitored by ultrasound scans.

6
Drug treatments

Many doctors still think that the best way to deal with troublesome fibroids is by surgery. But they do increasingly recognize that drugs have an important part to play in fibroid treatment. A common view currently among doctors is that drugs can buy you time, but that you will ultimately need surgery. If your problem is heavy, possibly painful, periods, it's certainly worth talking to your doctor about drug treatments.

Sally's story

Forty-year-old Sally discovered ten years ago that she had a fibroid. 'I was having an abortion and the doctors discovered that I had a fibroid the size of an orange pressing into one of my Fallopian tubes and also the ovary. This must have been the reason why sex had been getting rather painful. I had an operation to remove the fibroid. Everything was fine until about a year ago, when my periods became increasingly heavy and very painful. I had my coil removed but I kept on bleeding very badly, so I was referred to a gynaecologist. I had an abdominal ultrasound scan and was told I had another little fibroid, about 2 cm wide, in my womb-lining. The doctors suggested a hormonal coil to try and stop the bleeding, but my GP said it might not suit me because of my previous problems with the coil.

'At one point, I wanted to have a hysterectomy because the bleeding was so bad. When my mother's fibroids were discovered 20 years ago, the doctors immediately whipped out her womb. But my doctors say I'm too young to have a hysterectomy, and that I should try and cope with drug treatments. They want me, if possible, to go through a natural menopause and they think the little fibroid shouldn't cause me too many problems.

'When the bleeding was very bad I used to flood for about five days. One day I went through 40 super-plus tampons. I was having to take a day off work each month because of my periods, and was finding it very hard to manage my demanding job. I was also becoming anaemic and getting increasingly tired.

'For the last three months I've been on a drug called Cyklokapron. The flooding only lasts two days now and I've stopped passing the clots which were causing so much pain – I felt as though I was giving birth at one point. I also take Ibuprofen for the pain. I feel I can cope at the moment, but I'll see how things go. If my periods become awful again I may need to have a hysterectomy.'

Most of the women I spoke to didn't know much about drug options – though there are now more drug treatments which may help relieve period problems. Drugs may be the answer if they can control bleeding and pain successfully, without giving you distressing side-effects. If one drug doesn't work, talk to your doctor about trying another type of drug. It really is worth experimenting. Doctors do have their own preferences, based on their experience of treating women – but most doctors are willing to prescribe other drugs. You may, depending on the drug, need to persevere with several months of treatment for the maximum effect. If you are particularly keen on trying to cope with your symptoms by using drug treatments, try to see a doctor who is also interested in this approach and so therefore likely to be knowledgeable about the various drugs. Ask your doctor about the possibility of being referred to a hospital which has a menorrhagia clinic (which treats women suffering from heavy menstrual bleeding): doctors there may be particularly expert in drug treatments for fibroid problems.

Always ask about the side-effects of each drug, how it should be taken (for example, before or after a meal), and whether the drug could interact with any other drugs or over-the-counter products you are taking. Your doctor will work out the drug dosage and how long you should take the medicine. This advice may change if you have any side-effects, or if the drug is not working. As long as the drugs provide symptom-relief, it doesn't matter whether or not they shrink the fibroids, provided the fibroids aren't causing serious pressure problems. One group of drugs can shrink fibroids for a time – these are discussed at the end of this chapter.

The question of medical control of heavy bleeding may be of particular interest for women nearing the menopause, who are hoping to avoid surgery.

Sarah's story

Sarah was told by two gynaecologists that she should have a

hysterectomy. But she was anxious to avoid this operation if at all possible. 'I was given these pills which successfully controlled my bouts of very heavy bleeding within 24 hours. I then tried another drug treatment. I took pills for a number of days, and when I stopped taking them I had a bleed: I did this when the weekend was coming up, so I could be at home to cope with the flooding. The drug worked very well, though I was worried about some eye symptoms and tingling sensations in my arm at one point. I think I may be at the menopause now. I've decided not to take the pills any more as my last period was fairly light. Since then I've been fine, and have had no periods now for several months – just the odd hot flush.'

Non steroidal anti-inflammatory drugs (NSAIDs)

NSAIDs are the first line of treatment for heavy and painful periods. They work by blocking the activity of naturally produced, hormone-like chemicals called prostaglandins. These chemicals occur in many different body-tissues, and can cause a number of symptoms, including pain, inflammation and contraction of the womb-muscle. Women with heavy, painful periods seem to have more of these chemicals. NSAIDs can help by blocking the activity of the prostaglandins. The result is less pain and bleeding.

Drugs in this group include aspirin and ibuprofen preparations, available over the counter from your pharmacy. They can have side-effects, so always check individual drug labels. The sorts of side-effects are listed below under Ponstan.

Ponstan

Mefenamic acid (Ponstan) is a stronger type of NSAID available on prescription. Research shows that it can effectively cut down bleeding by up to 30 per cent in some women. Ponstan has a reputation as an effective and safe drug with few side-effects, which can reduce bleeding and also ease pain. You only need take the drug during your period. It works particularly well if taken a day or two before bleeding starts, because it more effectively blocks the build-up of prostaglandins. It's often prescribed three times a day, but one gynaecologist commented that it works best if taken four times a day. If you forget a dose, it is less effective.

However, some doctors argue that Ponstan is not helpful when heavy bleeding is caused by fibroids, though it can help with painful periods.

Louise's story

Louise found that Ponstan didn't control her symptoms. 'I was flooding and having dreadful cramps so I changed from taking Panadol to Ponstan. But my symptoms were too bad and it didn't work.'

Ponstan may cause stomach upsets – minimize the risk by taking it after food. You shouldn't take the drug if you have:

- an allergy to aspirin or other NSAIDs;
- severe kidney disease;
- a peptic ulcer;
- digestive disorders, including inflammatory bowel disease.

The drug can occasionally cause drowsiness or dizziness. Check with your doctor or pharmacist about taking other drugs or over-the-counter products with it. There may, for example, be problems if you take it together with lithium (a drug used to treat recurrent depression). Avoid alcohol, as it may increase the risk of stomach bleeding. If you develop severe diarrhoea, a skin rash, bloody or black tarry stools or vomit blood, see your doctor straightaway.

Cyklokapron

Tranexamic acid (Cyklokapron) works by improving the clotting mechanisms in the womb. There were worries initially that the drug might cause clotting elsewhere in the body, but this doesn't seem to happen in healthy women. But you shouldn't take this drug if you have a history of clotting disorders.

Cyklokapron is also taken during your period, but doesn't relieve period pains. Research shows that it can reduce bleeding by 50 per cent in some cases. However, it may be less effective if you have fibroids – though it's still worth trying. One study from Finland found that the drug didn't help women whose bleeding was caused by fibroids. However, the drug did reduce bleeding when there was no obvious cause for the heavy periods. For best effect, take four times a day. It can, however, increase the passage of clots which may increase pain (though in Sally's case, described above, it seems to have had the opposite effect).

Possible side-effects include nausea, vomiting, diarrhoea and giddiness. Another drug which works in the same way, and which has been used more recently is called ethamsylate (Dicynene). Possible side-effects again include nausea, vomiting and diarrhoea.

You may find that drugs such as Ponstan or Cyklokapron are all you need. However, even though they can substantially reduce bleeding, they may not be sufficient in some cases. As one gynaecologist pointed out, you are still losing a lot of blood if your blood-loss is reduced from 300 ml to 150 ml, as the definition of heavy bleeding is 80 ml.

The contraceptive Pill

Another possibility is the contraceptive Pill.

Jill's story

Jill found the Pill helpful. 'I took the combined Pill for ten years after I had an operation to remove my fibroids. It was wonderful, and I had hardly any bleeding.'

The combined Pill contains oestrogen and progestogen, and in effect produces a state of false pregnancy. It works by inhibiting the production of FSH and LH by the pituitary gland (as described in Chapter 2). As a result, the ovaries stop producing eggs. The combined Pill also thins the womb-lining. Research suggests that the combined Pill can significantly reduce bleeding in 90 per cent of women.

As discussed in Chapter 3, there is evidence that, if you have taken the combined Pill for ten years or so, you may be less likely to develop fibroids. Quite why this should be is unclear. The evidence suggests that pills with a higher amount of progestogen offset the effects of oestrogen. Progestogens (of which there are various types) are the synthetic equivalent of the natural female hormone progesterone. Progestogens have been developed because progesterone breaks down too rapidly to have much effect when taken by mouth. Oestrogen thickens the womb-lining, but progestogen thins and shrinks it, offsetting the effects of oestrogen.

In a natural cycle the two hormones are not balanced in the same way as with the combined Pill. As we have seen, oestrogen dominates in the first part of the cycle, while progesterone dominates in the second part. Taking a constant dose of the two hormones in the artificial cycle may help protect against fibroids developing, as oestrogen is constantly balanced by progestogen. The Pill may also slow fibroid growth.

But can the Pill help relieve symptoms, or affect fibroid size, if you already have fibroids which are causing heavy bleeding and perhaps pain? The Pill is usually very helpful in making periods lighter and reducing pain, as ovulation does not occur and the womb-lining is thinner. In the past there were fears that the Pill could make fibroids grow. But this was at a time when higher, 50 mg doses of oestrogen were used in the Pill – nowadays lower dosages of 30 mg are normally used. Fibroids may occasionally increase in size with the low-dose Pills, but it's unclear whether the Pill is responsible for the growth or whether the fibroids would have grown anyway.

Current advice is that if you have fibroids, you can take the low-dose, combined Pill, provided your symptoms do not worsen while you are on it. Some doctors think that problems can be minimized by a Pill which is high in progestogen. But there is no universal agreement on this point, and advice from one expert was to take the low-dose oestrogen and progestogen Pill in order to minimize the risk of side-effects from either of the two hormones.

If you do take the Pill, the fibroids should be carefully monitored with ultrasound scans. However, one expert pointed out that the Pill may not be so effective at relieving symptoms of heavy bleeding and pain caused by fibroids. In Jill's case (described above) the Pill was an effective treatment for a long time, but eventually she started to spot and then the heavy bleeding returned.

It is certainly worth talking to your doctor about trying it out as a treatment. Apart from the fibroids being checked, you will need to be carefully monitored because of other possible side-effects. Oestrogen increases the risk of abnormal blood clots in the body, though lower doses of oestrogen in the Pill have reduced this risk. Other possible side-effects include high blood-pressure, jaundice and liver disease, weight-gain and breast tenderness.

You shouldn't take the Pill if you:

• have high blood-pressure;

- smoke and are over 35;
- have a history of blood-clotting disorders;
- have (or have had) liver disease;
- suffer from severe migraine;
- have unexplained vaginal bleeding.

If you can't take the combined Pill for some reason, you may be able to take the progestogen-only Pill. It works mainly by thickening the fluid at the neck of the womb, making it harder for sperm to travel into the womb. It also makes the womb-lining less likely to accept a fertilized egg. Fewer women have taken this type of Pill, so less is known about its effects on the body generally. You can take this type of Pill if you have fibroids – but again, it may not be very helpful for relieving troublesome fibroid symptoms, and, according to one expert, is certainly no better than the combined Pill at relieving fibroid symptoms. It may also cause breakthrough bleeding, and sometimes small cysts on the ovaries – though these usually disappear.

To summarize: the low-dose combined Pill is unlikely to make fibroids grow. The combined Pill can be used to treat period problems, though it may be less effective when those problems are due to fibroids.

The Mirena coil

Mirena is a type of contraceptive coil which became available in this country for contraceptive purposes in 1995. The ordinary, copper-containing IUDs (intrauterine devices) have a reputation for causing pain and heavy bleeding during periods. But research shows that Mirena, called an intrauterine system, actually reduces bleeding substantially.

The Mirena coil mainly works by releasing a tiny amount of progestogen directly into the womb. The womb-lining becomes so thin that an embryo cannot implant properly in it. Periods become less painful and also much lighter, because there is hardly any womb-lining to shed. About one in five women stop having periods altogether. But, as with any contraceptive method, there are disadvantages – these include irregular bleeding and spotting for the first three months after insertion, and sometimes longer. Some doctors have said they have had to remove the Mirena because of this problem. There are few side-effects from the progestogen, because it acts locally on the womb-lining rather than throughout the body. But possible side-effects include headaches, depression, breast tenderness and small ovarian cysts which usually clear up.

At the moment, Mirena is licensed for contraceptive use – but research is underway into its use as a treatment for heavy periods. Research into Mirena as a treatment for fibroid problems is limited – though one study suggested it may be helpful.

It's worth inquiring about Mirena if you're happy about having a coil inserted. However, several doctors were keen to emphasize that Mirena may not work so well if the womb is distorted, due to the presence of submucous fibroids in the womb-lining. If there's a greatly increased surface area, the progestogen may be less effective at thinning the womb-lining. It may also be difficult to get the coil into the right place if the womb is very distorted. There is also a risk that the coil could be accidentally pushed through the womb-wall, as well as a higher risk that it could be expelled. One clinic which deals with heavy bleeding-problems is using certain drugs (which are discussed at the end of this chapter) to shrink the fibroids and return the womb to a normal shape; the Mirena coil is then inserted to try and keep the fibroids small and the womb-lining thin.

Progestogens

At one time, it was hoped that progestogens might be a useful treatment for fibroids, as they are often used in the treatment of heavy bleeding generally. The theory is that progestogens may help if you are not ovulating and producing progesterone in the second half of the cycle. But (as already mentioned) research shows that norethisterone, the progestogen most commonly prescribed by GPs for heavy periods, is in fact the least effective one at reducing heavy bleeding. However, it can help make cycles more regular. Progestogens also have side-effects which can include weight-gain, mood changes and swelling of the lower abdomen due to fluid retention.

But the most important point is that fibroid experts generally say that progestogen treatment is not usually effective when fibroids are largely responsible for heavy bleeding. There's also no evidence that progestogens shrink fibroids despite their anti-oestrogenic action. As discussed in Chapter 2, there's also now research which suggests that they may promote fibroid growth – though this is contentious. So the role of progestogen treatment for fibroids is confused. One specialist, however, says that progestogens may help if heavy bleeding is mainly caused by a lack of progesterone in anovulatory cycles, rather than by fibroids. These cycles, in which no egg is produced, are more common in women coming up to the menopause – but this is also the time when fibroids can be particularly troublesome. It may be difficult to know what is really causing the problem, and may explain why Susan, 44, found norethisterone helpful when she took it two years ago.

Susan's story

'I was getting a lot of period pain and bleeding, so I went to hospital and had a scan which revealed that I had a 4 cm fibroid in my womb-lining. I took norethisterone for nine months. My periods became more regular and not so heavy, though I still had lots of pain. But I stopped taking the drug because I didn't want to take hormonal treatment for any length of time.'

So it's worth talking to your doctor about progestogen treatment for heavy bleeding, if nothing else has worked. It's also accepted that at high doses, progestogens can help with a sudden, torrential bout of uncontrollable bleeding (a high dose of oestrogen can also stop bleeding, but doctors do not usually use this treatment in this country). A dose of up to 30 mg of norethisterone usually stops the bleeding in 24–48 hours, according to one doctor. The dose is then reduced and finally stopped over the next few days, when another lighter bleed usually occurs. The progestogen seems to work by stabilizing the womb-lining and shrinking the blood-vessels in that area. However, high doses should not be given on a long-term basis because of possible side-effects, such as heart disease.

Danazol

Danazol (brand name Danol) is sometimes used to treat fibroids. It is a synthetic hormone derived from the male hormone testosterone. Danazol produces a false menopause in the body, which is reversible once the drug is stopped. The drug interferes with the basic control of the menstrual cycle. It lowers levels of oestrogen and progesterone in the body by blocking production of the FSH and LH hormones produced by the pituitary gland (see Chapter 2). It is effective at lessening blood-loss, but again there's less research into how effective it is when fibroids are present. The theory is that, because it reduces oestrogen-levels, it may shrink fibroids – but there is little research on this. At high doses it may shrink fibroids a bit: one study reported that fibroids reduced in size by only about 20 per cent when a daily dose of 800 mg was taken for six months. The newer GnRH drugs, discussed at the end of this chapter, reduced fibroids far more effectively.

But apart from the question of whether or not it shrinks fibroids, danazol can stop periods altogether, or significantly reduce bleeding depending on the dosage used. However, if taking danazol, you should also use an effective non-hormonal contraceptive, as ovulation may occur at a low dosage, and the drug can cause foetal abnormalities. The drug is not very widely used in the treatment of fibroids, mainly because of its unpleasant side-effects. It can produce male characteristics – such as a deep voice, acne and excessive hair-growth. Other side-effects include weight-gain, headaches, nausea, dizziness, muscle cramps, hot flushes, mood changes and depression. As a result, only short courses of the drug are usually prescribed.

However, one gynaecologist argues that the drug can be helpful if given in lower doses. At 200 mg daily, the drug has fewer side-effects and is better tolerated. He prescribes it for six months to a year, and uses it particularly for intramural fibroids which are causing period problems. At this dosage, most women keep having light periods. Women also still have some oestrogen, and so do not suffer from the possible loss of bone-density that may occur at higher doses. Problems may be kept in check for a time once drug-treatment is stopped.

However, even at this low dosage, danazol may cause harmful circulatory changes by increasing levels of fats in the blood while lowering protective cholesterol levels. It may also affect liver function. So it's important that you are monitored carefully while on the drug. Some women also find that 200 mg is insufficient to control bleeding, but that higher doses can produce intolerable side-effects, as already mentioned.

You shouldn't take the drug if, for instance, you suffer from a blood-clotting disorder, have heart, kidney or liver failure or have abnormal vaginal bleeding.

Gestrinone

Gestrinone (brand-name Dimetriose) is similar to danazol, but needs to be taken only once or twice a week and can be taken for up to a year. There is some research which shows this drug only slightly reduces fibroid size. However, when you're on this drug your periods will stop or become infrequent – so it can control heavy bleeding, but it's not used long-term. After treatment, some women find their symptoms do not return, while others do have recurring symptoms. There are fewer side-effects with this drug than with danazol: it's less likely to cause excessive hair-growth or deepen the voice, and has a less harmful effect on cholesterol levels. As with danazol, you must not become pregnant while on this drug.

Tamoxifen

In the past, tamoxifen was sometimes used to reduce heavy bleeding. In one study, 20 mg a day was given for three months to six pre-menopausal women. Fibroids did not significantly reduce in size after six months, but most women said their periods were lighter. Again, it's not intended that tamoxifen should be taken long term. However, most gynaecologists nowadays are unlikely to prescribe tamoxifen, because it causes polyps and increases the risk of cancer of the womb-lining.

GnRH (gonadotrophin releasing hormone) analogues

GnRH analogues (sometimes called luteinizing hormone releasing hormone analogues) are called analogues because they are rather like the natural gonadotrophin releasing hormone in structure. They overstimulate the pituitary gland so that it eventually stops producing FSH and LH – the two hormones which are essential for ovulation. The ovaries stop producing oestrogen, which leads to a temporary menopause. Periods usually start about eight weeks after stopping treatment, but occasionally may not start up again.

The two GnRH drugs often used are buserelin and goserelin. They are not taken by mouth because they break down too fast in the body to have any effect. They are taken either by nasal spray, which you have to sniff several times a day, or by a monthly injection. Alternatively, a local anaesthetic is used to insert a monthly implant just underneath the skin. A barrier contraceptive should be used while you are on the drug. Some women may not be able to take these drugs because they are allergic to them.

When they became available in the 1980s, these drugs were hailed as the answer to troublesome fibroids. They are the only drugs which reliably relieve symptoms. They stop bleeding problems and relieve pelvic pain. The GnRH analogues also shrink fibroids – even large ones – by about 50 per cent. Reduction in size normally occurs in the first three months of a treatment cycle, which is usually six months long.

However, there are drawbacks to these drugs. They are usually only taken for six months because of their side-effects, such as hot flushes. If taken for a longer time, they cause a number of other important side-effects, such as mood swings, depression, vaginal dryness and in particular bone-thinning. They can also raise cholesterol levels and reduce levels of protective cholesterol in the body. Any bone-density loss is reversible – though it may not be if you take the drug for longer than six months. Once you stop taking the drugs, the fibroids regrow to their original size within about three months, and symptoms usually return. If you are underweight your doctor may think these drugs are unsuitable because of the bone-thinning they can cause. Instead, danazol may be prescribed for heavy bleeding. The drugs are also very expensive at the moment, costing over a £100 a month. As a result of all these things, the drugs are seen as a short-term option.

They are currently used in various ways. They may be prescribed for three months before surgery, to reduce fibroid size and blood-supply to the fibroids. Haemoglobin levels then have a chance to recover to normal if you're anaemic, because you're not losing blood each month. There's evidence that use of these drugs before surgery reduces blood-loss during the operation and that recovery time is faster. There is also a smaller risk of scarring occurring inside the abdomen, because of the smaller amount of blood-loss. This is an important consideration if you want to get pregnant later on, because scarring inside the abdomen can reduce your ability to conceive. Some surgeons also say it's easier to remove fibroids after drug treatment with GnRH analogues.

Louise's story

Louise took one of these drugs by monthly injection for three months before her operation to remove fibroids. 'I was warned about dire side-effects of the drug. But I was very lucky. I just had a few hot flushes. I had treatment for two months after the operation and my body was back to normal 50 days after the last drug treatment.'

Some doctors think that these drugs can tide you over to the menopause, if you are fairly near to it – at which point the fibroids should shrink naturally.

Addback therapy

Doctors are trying out various combinations of what is called addback therapy. This is done to protect against menopausal side-effects – in particular, bone-thinning. It's all highly experimental, but some doctors say that GnRH analogues, plus addback therapy, can be given for one to two years.

The idea is to give you just enough oestrogen to relieve symptoms, without encouraging fibroid regrowth. After three months of the GnRH analogue, a small amount of oestrogen is taken in addition to the analogue, to counter the menopausal side-effects produced by the analogue; sometimes a tiny amount of progestogen may also be given. According to one specialist this, rather than surgery, may be the answer for women who are in their late forties with medium-sized symptom-causing fibroids.

One study looked at five women who took GnRH drugs for three months and then continued to receive this, plus addback therapy. The women were studied for two years. Within three months womb-size had decreased by half. The women initially had hot flushes, but these stopped once they received the addback therapy and they suffered no bone-thinning.

But this approach is highly contentious. The effects of taking these powerful drugs for a long time are not known. It may not be a good idea to give powerful hormonal drugs, for a year or so, to women who are starting to go through significant hormonal changes as they approach the menopause. The long-term consequences of taking these drugs for a couple of years around the time of the menopause are just not known at the moment.

Summary

- Drugs have a role to play in the treatment of fibroid symptoms. But most doctors at the moment do not consider that drug treatments are an alternative to surgical treatments – though they may be in the future. However, drugs may see you through to the menopause, if you are near to it. Specialist heavy-bleeding clinics may be particularly helpful with drug treatments.

- Whether or not drug treatments are appropriate for you will depend on your symptoms and age, and on whether you want children. There are various drugs which can provide relief for heavy bleeding. They all have advantages and disadvantages. If one doesn't work, talk to your doctor about trying another one.
- If you want children, you may need to have the fibroids removed.
- Always ask about the side-effects of any treatment. If you want children, ask whether the drugs could make conception in the future more difficult. Ask whether the drug could interact with any other drug or over-the-counter product you are taking. Check how you should take it, and whether you should take additional contraceptive measures.

7

Surgical removal of fibroids

Despite advances in drug treatment, many doctors think that the best treatment for troublesome fibroids is surgery, and that the best type of surgery is hysterectomy. However, doctors are prepared (though sometimes reluctantly) to consider just removing the fibroids – a procedure called myomectomy. This chapter looks at ways of doing this. The various types of hysterectomy are covered in the next chapter.

As discussed in Chapter 5, your consent to surgery is needed, if you and your doctor have decided that surgery is the right option. To recap:

- Ask your doctor to explain the advantages and disadvantages of the procedure, such as complications and side-effects.
- Ask whether there are any alternative surgical options.
- Ask how effective the operation is, and what it entails – for example, how long you will be in hospital and how you'll feel afterwards.
- It can sometimes be helpful to talk to women who have had the operation to find out what it is like from a woman's perspective.
- There is always a risk that surgery can cause infection and damage to body-tissue. Minor post-operative complications are common, though fortunately more serious ones are rare.

Some sort of surgery may be necessary if you fall into any of the following groups:

1 If drugs cannot control the severe bleeding and pain.
2 If you have serious pressure symptoms, for example a fibroid pressing on the urinary system.
3 If a fibroid is causing fertility problems.
4 If the fibroid is cancerous, in which case a hysterectomy will be needed; the fibroid will have to be removed and inspected if it appears cancerous, though it can be biopsied in a less invasive way at a few hospitals (as discussed in Chapter 4).

Myomectomy means the removal of fibroids – a procedure which was first performed in the last century. Nowadays there are various ways of removing fibroids surgically, as new techniques have been developed. Gynaecologists all have their own preferences, based on their experience, and will carry out the procedure in slightly different ways. Once the fibroid has been taken out, it is checked in the laboratory to see if it's cancerous. Women are not always offered the option of myomectomy.

Lucy's story

> About four years ago, when Lucy was 49, she asked if she could have her fibroids removed. She was told this was only possible for women who wanted to have children, and that myomectomy was never offered to women in their forties. The only sort of surgery she was offered was hysterectomy.

Clearly there may sometimes be good reasons why certain medical procedures are not advisable. But this isn't always so. See if you can be referred to another hospital if your hospital appears to have a standard policy that older women who have completed their families cannot have a myomectomy.

Hysteroscopic myomectomy

The technique of hysteroscopic myomectomy is suitable for removing small, submucous fibroids, usually less than 2.5 cm wide, which are underneath the womb-lining or which are hanging into the womb-cavity on a stalk. If your problem is heavy bleeding, and your doctor thinks this is caused by submucous fibroids, then the simplest solution may be to remove them. Your doctor may also advise you to have them removed if you want to get pregnant. It can be a relatively quick, simple way of removing the fibroids.

Angela's story

> Angela had a hysteroscopic myomectomy after being advised to have a submucous fibroid removed because it might be interfering with her fertility. 'I wasn't allowed to eat anything after midnight, and went in the following day for surgery as a day case. I was given a light anaesthetic, and after the operation spent the rest of the day

71

sleeping. I went home later on, and was back to normal within about a week. I had slight pelvic cramps and bleeding for a couple of days.'

During the procedure, the neck of the womb is widened slightly and a tiny viewing-instrument, the hysteroscope, is carefully inserted into the womb. During surgery, fluid is pushed into and out of the womb through the hysteroscope, so that the gynaecologist can see inside the womb properly. Various instruments can be inserted through the hysteroscope to destroy or cut out the fibroids. For example, a laser can be used to cut the fibroids up in slices, or to nip off fibroids on stalks. Carbon dioxide lasers have traditionally been used for gynaecological surgery – but neodymium:YAG (Nd:YAG) lasers are proving more useful for treating fibroids. This type of laser seals as it cuts, which is an advantage because of the risk of bleeding-problems with fibroids. Alternatively, a wire loop, called a resectoscope, is used to cut out the fibroids.

Hysteroscopic myomectomy has various advantages. There are no abdominal incisions, so recovery is fast – and there is usually little scarring within the abdomen. Research suggests that it is a good treatment. But fibroids can regrow, and symptoms may return. In one study of 94 women who had this procedure using the resectoscope, 23 women started getting symptoms again and 15 of them needed further surgery. As mentioned, results are even better if the Nd:YAG laser is used.

As with any surgical procedure there are risks – though in skilled hands this is thought to be a safe procedure. About 50 per cent of gynaecologists should be able to carry out this procedure, according to one expert.

Larger submucous fibroids

Hysteroscopic myomectomy is not always a simple procedure – for example, if the womb is very distorted. Also, if the fibroid is deeply embedded in the womb-wall, there is a risk that the womb-wall could be perforated as the surgeon tries to remove the fibroid. The womb-wall might rupture in a subsequent pregnancy if it's perforated during hysteroscopic myomectomy. According to one study, this happened to four per cent of women.

Experts in hysteroscopic myomectomy, however, do use the

technique for larger submucous fibroids which may be deeply embedded in the womb-wall. GnRH drugs are used for three months before the operation to shrink the fibroids, which are then removed. You should use a barrier method of contraception if you're taking these drugs, to make sure there is no chance of pregnancy. During the operation, the surgeon may use a laparoscope to view the womb-wall from the other side, to make sure it's not perforated.

Some experts use a two-step procedure (that is, two hysteroscopic myomectomies) to remove embedded fibroids. Step one involves removing as much as possible of the fibroids. GnRH drugs are then taken for three months. Step two involves removing the rest of the fibroids. Again, gynaecologists use variations on this method.

One gynaecologist says it's possible to remove a fibroid up to 5 cm wide in one step. GnRH drugs are taken beforehand. During the operation, the visible part of the fibroid is removed. The deeper part of the fibroid then becomes visible and can be removed as it is pushed outwards by contractions of the womb-wall.

Infertility

If your doctor suggests that submucous fibroids may be making you infertile, consider getting a second opinion from a fertility specialist. It may be that the fibroids aren't responsible for your infertility, and if you have the procedure, you run the risk of infection entering the pelvis and increasing your fertility problems. There is no easy answer to this. Doctors will have different views depending on their experience.

Angela's story

Angela's experience demonstrates this. A fertility specialist advised her to have her submucous fibroids removed. 'After I'd had it done, I consulted another fertility specialist who suggested that it wasn't necessary to have had this done. It's several years since I had the operation and I'm still not pregnant.'

The operation

Hysteroscopic myomectomy is usually performed on an outpatient basis (that is, you don't need an overnight stay), and is normally done under general anaesthetic. You may be able to have a local anaesthetic, which can be injected into the neck of the womb, plus a sedative. Ask

73

about this if you're very worried about having a general anaesthetic. There is always a risk of death associated with having a general anaesthetic – but this is very small. You are far more likely to be run over crossing a road than to suffer a major complication as a result of having a general anaesthetic. General anaesthetics are much safer today than they were in the past. It's now common for anaesthetists to give several drugs to minimize the risk of side-effects. A pre-med is usually given to calm you, then a combination of drugs is given before and during the operation, often by injection. Sometimes anaesthetic gases are inhaled.

You'll need to rest afterwards in the recovery room for several hours, for the effects of the anaesthetic or sedative to wear off. Painkillers will be given as necessary, but you shouldn't have too much discomfort. Expect to feel fragile after the operation. You may feel dizzy and vomit, but should recover from any hangover effects in a few days. Don't drive for 24 hours afterwards and avoid alcohol for a few days.

You may be back to normal in a day or so, but some women need longer. Expect to have a watery, blood-stained discharge for a few days. Use sanitary pads rather than tampons, which may increase the risk of infection moving upwards from the vagina. If you have very heavy bleeding, acute pain or a bad-smelling vaginal discharge, see your doctor immediately in case there is an infection. You can make love again as soon as you feel comfortable. The gynaecologist will check how you are about six weeks after the operation.

Endometrial resection or ablation

If you don't want children or have completed your family, your gynaecologist may suggest removing the womb-lining at the same time as taking out the fibroids. Some (though not all) gynaecologists think that removal of the lining may also help prevent fibroids regrowing, because growth-factors are removed.

If you have your womb-lining removed, you become infertile – though there is still a possibility of an embryo implanting in the womb. You need to keep on using contraception after this procedure because of this possibility. If a pregnancy were to start developing it could be dangerous for you and the baby.

There are now various ways of removing the womb-lining. The

main methods involve using either a resectoscope to remove it or a laser to destroy it. If the lining is taken out with a wire, samples can be sent to a laboratory to check for cancer if there are worries about this. You may be given drugs beforehand to help shrink the womb-lining. Alternatively, the operation may be done immediately after a period, when the lining is thinner.

Removing the womb-lining is a relatively minor procedure – but it carries risks, so discuss these with your gynaecologist (you could just opt to have the submucous fibroids out). If the surgeon cuts or burns too deeply, the womb-wall could be perforated, with possible damage to other organs such as the bladder or bowel. Research also suggests that some women may experience increasing pelvic pain after the womb-lining is removed.

It is likely that small parts of the womb-lining may be left behind afterwards. If you are near the menopause and want to have HRT (hormone replacement therapy), you will be advised to take combined oestrogen/progestogen therapy. The progestogen part of the HRT will prevent cancer of the womb-lining developing.

If you have the combined procedure, recovery time is the same as for hysteroscopic myomectomy. Bleeding may continue for a week, and possibly for up to six or so weeks afterwards. After about four months, most women will have stopped bleeding altogether or have regular, light periods. When the womb-lining is removed, periods stop in about 50 per cent of women; 40 per cent still have light periods, but about 10 per cent of women continue bleeding heavily and will need further surgery. There's little research into how well the procedure works for women who have had fibroids.

Abdominal myomectomy by laparotomy

This is done to remove intramural and subserous fibroids. If you have a mixture of the various types of fibroids, the surgeon may use this operation to remove all of them. But it's possible the surgeon may want to do a two-step procedure, using a hysteroscope to take out the submucous fibroids and then performing an abdominal myomectomy for the other types of fibroids.

An abdominal myomectomy is the conventional way of removing fibroids, through a large incision in the abdomen. This type of operation is called a laparotomy. Abdominal myomectomy has been performed for many years, but some women are still not given information about this procedure, according to one adviser on health problems. They are only told about having a hysterectomy.

In the past, abdominal myomectomy was offered only to women who wanted to have children. But doctors increasingly recognize that some women who have finished childbearing also want a myomectomy rather than a hysterectomy.

Ruth's story

Ruth, 50, had her only child when she was 30. 'When I was in my mid-forties, and was having a cervical smear done, the doctor said he thought I had a fibroid. I was told not to worry about it, but over the next few years I started going to the loo more often. My abdomen was bloated, though there was no change in my periods, which were fine. But my stomach was getting bigger and I could actually feel the fibroid through my stomach-wall. I was eventually referred to a gynaecologist who did an ultrasound scan and found a fibroid the size of a 19-week pregnancy. He said I should have my womb out, but I didn't want to have this done because I felt fine apart from the fibroid. So I had a second opinion, and this other gynaecologist also recommended a hysterectomy. I didn't want a hysterectomy unless it was absolutely necessary – on the other hand, I could no longer lead a normal life. I was going to the loo all the time, almost living in the bathroom. There was a great cloud hanging over my life.

'After checking around I found an expert who was prepared to try and just remove the fibroid. He warned me, however, that he might have to remove the whole womb if there were complications. But the operation was a success.'

The operation

Before the operation you may be given GnRH drugs to shrink the fibroids and reduce their blood-supply – though this depends on the gynaecologist's view of whether the drugs will make the operation easier. The gynaecologist decided that the drugs were not necessary in Ruth's case (above). If you take the drugs, remember that you should also keep using some other form of contraceptive. If you've been losing a lot of blood and are anaemic, the gynaecologist may also want you to take the GnRH drugs to stop your periods. This allows your haemoglobin-levels to return to normal before the operation. You may need a blood transfusion before the operation, if you are very anaemic.

The operation involves shelling out the growths from the capsules in which they grow. You will be given a general anaesthetic as it's a major operation. A low abdominal cut along the bikini-line is usually made – though a vertical incision may be necessary if the fibroid is very large. The fibroids are removed from their capsules with a hot wire, surgical knife or laser. As discussed above, the Nd:YAG laser can reduce blood-loss and also post-operative pain. Sometimes the equivalent of a corkscrew is used to pull out the fibroids. Once the fibroids are removed, the empty capsules are closed with stitches.

Possible complications and consequences

A myomectomy is a more complex operation than a hysterectomy, which is why gynaecologists have not been in favour of doing it. Fibroids have a big blood-supply, and when they are removed can bleed a lot. If bleeding cannot be controlled, the gynaecologist may have to do a hysterectomy – though this should rarely happen nowadays. The operation can also take a long time if there are lots of fibroids to scoop out. Ideally, only the ones which cause symptoms should be removed – though this can be difficult for the gynaecologist to assess. It's important to remove the fibroids with the minimum amount of damage to the womb-wall. This will depend on the skill of the surgeon, as well as how deeply embedded the fibroids are, and how many need to be removed. As with all surgery, there is a risk of death – though this is low for myomectomy, at under one per cent.

If you're hoping to get pregnant after the operation, it's important that your womb can cope with a pregnancy and not rupture: too much tunnelling can substantially weaken the womb-wall. One expert removed 107 fibroids in one operation – mostly tiny lumps, plus some large ones; the woman subsequently got pregnant and carried the baby successfully. Doctors may, however, want to do a Caesarean to prevent problems occurring during labour, because the womb-wall may not be strong enough.

The risk of infection is also high after this operation. One gynaecologist, who is very experienced in performing the operation, explained that it's important to have a drain in the pelvis for a couple of days afterwards to prevent pools of blood forming in the pelvis. An antibiotic is also given, to prevent an infection developing.

Fibroids can also regrow after the operation. In a large study of 600 women who had the operation between 1970 and 1984, fibroids regrew in 27 per cent of women. There's no evidence that certain types of fibroids are more likely to regrow. But women who only had one fibroid had a smaller chance of fibroid regrowth. Women who had a baby after the myomectomy were also less likely to have further fibroid problems. It's also important to repeat the point made to me by one doctor: if fibroids do regrow, they may not necessarily cause problems.

Problems caused by adhesions

As after any gynaecological surgery, adhesions can form. Adhesions are the joining together of normally unconnected body parts by bands of fibrous tissue, the result of scarring after inflammation or injury in the pelvic area. Scar-tissue can stick pelvic organs together, and make a subsequent hysterectomy much more difficult.

If you want to get pregnant, it's important to be aware that it may be more difficult if scar-tissue blocks the opening to the Fallopian tubes. This would prevent the egg being wafted down the tube.

Gynaecologists try to minimize the risk of adhesions developing by stopping any bleeding, by trying to prevent infection developing, and by washing out the abdominal cavity with certain solutions to prevent blood-clots forming.

Conclusion

It's always very important to find out how experienced the gynaecologist is in myomectomy techniques. In experienced hands and with the latest surgical techniques and drugs, the operation carries far fewer risks. It's very unlikely that the operation would turn into a hysterectomy, but the gynaecologist can never know beforehand quite how the operation is going to go. If you do not want a hysterectomy, then discuss this issue carefully with your gynaecologist.

Preparing for abdominal myomectomy

* It's worth trying to get into a good state of health for the operation. If you're very overweight, you may be asked to lose excess weight. Healing takes longer, and the risk of infection is greater if you are carrying too much weight.
* Sometimes a blood transfusion is necessary before surgery, if you are very anaemic. If you are anaemic, make sure you talk to your

doctor about iron supplements to make sure you are ready to cope with surgery, so that you don't need a blood transfusion. The GnRH drugs may be sufficient to allow your blood-count to improve, but you may also need additional supplements.

- If you lose a lot of blood during the operation, you may also need a blood transfusion. There is a higher risk of this happening in this operation than in a hysterectomy, so it's worth talking to your doctor about an autologous blood transfusion – that is, when your blood is collected before the operation, so that if necessary it can be used during surgery (rather than your having blood from someone else). A pint of your blood would be taken each week for several weeks, and stored in readiness for the operation. But the blood can only be stored for five weeks, so the date when you start self-donation will depend on the date of the operation. But this isn't always known or can change. You need to be healthy and not anaemic in order to self-donate.

  The disadvantage of using other people's blood is that it lowers your immunity. This means that you have an increased risk of getting an infection. If you use your own blood you are less likely to get a post-operative infection, and you may end up leaving hospital a few days earlier. But only a limited number of UK hospitals currently offer this service: talk to your gynaecologist if you are interested in this possibility.

- If you smoke, try to stop before surgery. Smokers are more likely to develop blood-clots and chest infections after operations.

- You should stop taking the combined contraceptive Pill four weeks before the operation, and use another contraceptive method instead. The Pill can increase the risk of blood-clots forming. Get your doctor's guidance on this.

- Practise regular relaxation techniques beforehand (see Chapter 10 for more details). Patients who are very scared and nervy can take longer to recover from an operation. They may bleed more, and so have more infections and complications. If you're calm beforehand, you'll help yourself.

- Practise pelvic-floor exercises, as described in Chapter 10.

- You will not be able to have the operation if you are having your period. Let the hospital know if you are due to have one on the date set for the operation.

- The operation may also have to be cancelled if you are unwell or have an infection, as this could make surgery more risky.

After the operation

When you wake up, expect to have a sore, bruised abdomen. You will need sanitary protection for a few days. If you develop a smelly discharge, it's a sign of infection and you will need antibiotic treatment. Minor side-effects include coughs and chest infections, and a sore throat due to the tube which will have been put down your throat during the operation to help you breath, as you'll have been given a muscle relaxant. It's quite common for a blood-clot to form just under the surface of the skin. This often clears up on its own, though it sometimes need attention.

You may have a tube called a catheter inserted into your bladder to help you pass urine – though this may not be necessary. You may also find that you have a drain, a tube inserted through the skin next to the abdominal incision to remove blood collecting in the pelvis. This is left in place for a couple of days.

You will be encouraged to get up and walk as soon as you can, to minimize the risk of a blood-clot developing. While you are in bed, move your ankles round in a circle – first one way, then the other – to get your circulation moving, and also flex your ankles and knees. Repeat these movements at short regular intervals until you get back to normal walking. After an anaesthetic it's important to exercise your lungs. Take a deep, slow breath in through your nose, hold for a count of two and sigh as you breathe out. Repeat this several times. This exercise also helps loosen any phlegm which may have collected in your chest. Stitches will be removed after about seven days, and internal stitches should dissolve over the next couple of weeks.

You'll probably be allowed home after about a week. Allow about a month to get back to normal, and in the meantime treat yourself gently. You may feel tired at times, and rather depressed – but this is normal. Physiotherapists who specialize in gynaecology can give advice about exercises to help you regain your strength and improve muscle-tone in the abdominal area. The physiotherapist can also teach you how to do pelvic-floor exercises to tone up the muscles which support the pelvic organs. These exercises are described in Chapter 10. Ask when you can safely start doing the various exercises. The normal rule is as soon as possible, but start by doing a small amount of exercise and gradually build this up each day.

Your gynaecologist will check you about six weeks after the operation. If everything has healed up, you should then be able to make love if you want to. The abdominal incision may be sore for a while, so try out positions which don't put pressure on this area.

If you want to try for a baby, you'll probably be advised to wait for about three months to give the womb a chance to recover. It depends on what exactly was done to the womb-wall.

Angela's story

Angela had an abdominal myomectomy four years ago, in order to try and improve her fertility. 'I was scared stiff at the thought that, if the worst happened, I could lose my womb – but was told I needed to have the fibroid removed. I had to take a drug called goserelin for three months beforehand to shrink the fibroids. It wasn't a pleasant experience. I had awful night-sweats and mood swings, crying one minute and laughing the next.

'The operation was apparently a success, but I needed a blood transfusion. I was in hospital for about a week and then insisted on going home because I felt so well. I think I came through surgery pretty well because I'm fit. I don't smoke or drink, and I did exercises before the operation to make sure I was in good shape.

'On my first day back at home, my husband went off to work. I was on my own. I started to cry and cry. I think it was a release of emotions. I was so pleased that I still had my womb, that the operation was a success and that I didn't have cancer. But I also felt sad because I'd lost a part of myself, even though it was a fibroid. My sister stayed with me for a week, which helped.

'I was advised not to go back to work for at least eight weeks, but I returned after four weeks as I wanted to get back to normal. But I was hobbling round the office so I had to go home again and didn't return to work for another two weeks. I think I was driving myself very hard. I felt guilty that my colleagues were having to cover for me, though they were wonderful and didn't mind doing this. After about three months I was fine. My periods became a bit lighter, four as opposed to five days. That's the only difference I noticed. I've been monitored with scans regularly to check whether the fibroids have regrown. They haven't as far as I know, but I suspect they are regrowing. I think I'm just very anxious because I still haven't conceived and time is marching on.'

81

Infertility and abdominal myomectomy

If you are having an abdominal myomectomy to improve your fertility, there are several points to note. Your doctor should discuss these with you beforehand, so you can weigh up the risks properly.

- You could possibly end up having a hysterectomy because of complications – though this is very unlikely to happen, particularly if the surgeon is experienced in doing the operation.

Alison's story

Alison, 32, has had several miscarriages. She has been told that large fibroids are making it difficult for a baby to develop properly. She's been offered a myomectomy, but has decided against this for the time being. 'I've refused this at the moment' and I'm putting up with the heavy periods. I'm so worried that I might end up in a worse position if I have myomectomy because I risk losing my womb. I couldn't face the thought of never having my own child.'

- Any gynaecological procedure may increase fertility problems because of adhesions, which can block the entrance to the tubes. This could make conception more difficult.
- A myomectomy can weaken the womb-wall if lots of fibroids are removed, or if the fibroids were deeply embedded. This could affect a subsequent pregnancy.
- As discussed in Chapter 3, fibroids do not necessarily cause infertility, but they can do – and myomectomy may be the answer. In one study of 1,202 women, 40 per cent conceived after the operation. In another study, the miscarriage rate before myomectomy was 41 per cent – as opposed to 10 per cent after the operation. Get specialist advice from an infertility expert as to whether your fibroids are causing infertility – though, as we've seen, experts may well have different views.

Laparoscopic myomectomy

Some surgeons now do abdominal myomectomy using minimally invasive surgery, commonly called keyhole surgery. Instead of a major incision, tiny punctures are made in the abdomen. The operation is called a laparoscopic myomectomy (the basic technique is the same as for the diagnostic laparoscopy described in Chapter 4). A general anaesthetic is needed, and a one- or two-day stay in hospital.

Carbon dioxide is pumped into the abdomen, and a telescope called a laparoscope is inserted through an incision just underneath the navel. The laparoscope consists of a long tube with a series of lenses and a powerful light-source connected to a video camera. One or two other tiny incisions are made near the pubic hairline, through which various instruments are passed. A laser is normally used to remove the fibroids, as this reduces tissue damage. The fibroids are shelled out of their capsules, chopped up and placed in a special bag which is removed through one of the openings.

As a general rule, this type of myomectomy is only done if there are no more than four fibroids in the womb-wall. Each fibroid should be no more than 11 cm wide.

Recovery is much quicker than with other types of myomectomy, because the abdomen is punctured rather than cut. There is less scarring and tissue damage, and therefore less pain after this operation – whereas with the major incision made in a laparotomy, there is a lot of tissue trauma which takes time to heal, and you may feel unwell for several months afterwards.

However, keyhole surgery is more complicated, and can take a lot longer than other types of myomectomy, because of the tiny instruments which are used. Sewing up internal wounds and chopping up the fibroids with these miniature instruments can take a long time. It's difficult surgery, and the gynaecologist has to control bleeding in order to see properly with the special equipment. GnRH drugs are usually taken for three months beforehand to shrink the fibroids, which should make the operation easier and less bloody. If there is a lot of scar-tissue inside the abdomen, the gynaecologist may have to convert the operation into a conventional myomectomy. There is also a possibility that the surgeon may have to perform a hysterectomy because of complications.

After the operation, you'll find you have two or three small cuts, one just below the navel and one or two just around the pubic hairline. The incisions, covered by a transparent dressing, will have one or two stitches which should dissolve within about ten days. Due to the gas used, you may have some shoulder-pain for a couple of days (as explained on page 42). You may have some vaginal bleeding for a couple of weeks, so use sanitary pads rather than tampons to minimize the risk of infection. You can make love when you feel comfortable.

Helen's story

Helen had a conventional abdominal myomectomy 13 years ago, and more recently a laparoscopic myomectomy. 'After the first operation, I had to stay in hospital for two weeks. I felt as though I'd been kicked in the stomach by a horse. I had a 15-cm scar on my abdomen, and had to walk bent over double for the first week. For the next six weeks, I had to take it easy – I didn't make a full recovery for about six months.

'The fibroids regrew, and ten years later I had keyhole surgery to remove them. The growths were taken out through three 5-mm cuts in my abdomen. I had the operation one day and was out of hospital the next day. It was amazing. I had a bit of pain the first day, and then nothing more than a stinging feeling. Two weeks later I was back to normal.'

Louise's story

Louise also found recovery much quicker. She too had had a conventional operation some years ago. She has recently had a laparoscopic myomectomy. 'I was in hospital for 24 hours, and back to work in two weeks.'

Ruth's story

Ruth had keyhole surgery to remove her very large fibroid. It's not usually done for large fibroids – but the expert decided it was possible in her case. 'I had the operation done on a Monday. Afterwards there were four tiny incisions in my abdomen. I was home on Thursday, cleaning the house on Friday and back to work the next week.'

Summary

It's important to be aware of the following points if you want to have a laparoscopic myomectomy.

- It takes longer and is more complex than a conventional abdominal myomectomy.

- The surgeon has to use hand and eye co-ordination skills similar to those used in playing computer games. Make sure the surgeon is qualified to do this highly skilled surgery. In untrained hands the operation can be dangerous. There is the risk of damage to the bladder, bowel and ureters, the tubes coming from the kidneys to the bladder.

Questions to ask include:

- Am I suitable for this type of surgery? (If you've had previous abdominal surgery it may be difficult for the surgeon to see inside the abdomen properly because of the scar-tissue.)
- Has the surgeon lots of experience of doing this operation?
- How do the risks and complications of this operation compare to those of a conventional myomectomy?

Vaginal myomectomy

A few gynaecologists prefer, if possible, to remove intramural and subserous fibroids through the vagina. Again, GnRH drugs are given beforehand for three months, to shrink the fibroids. A small incision is made in the vagina, and the womb is pulled into the opening so that the fibroid can be shelled out. The womb is put back into its normal position and the incision sewn up.

Advantages include: no abdominal scars, and a quicker operation time, because standard-sized instruments can be used rather than the tiny ones used in a laparoscopic myomectomy. But the technique can't be done if the womb is more than the size of a 12–14 week pregnancy. As with any technique, it needs to be evaluated. If you want this done, ask about the risks and make sure that the surgeon is experienced in the technique. One specialist considered this operation out of date, and could see no reason to do it.

Myolysis

Myolysis, known as laser drilling, is being used in a few centres. It was first used in the late 1980s, and is still a highly experimental procedure not widely available. The technique deprives the fibroids of their blood-supply so that they wither and shrink. A general anaesthetic is needed for myolysis, which is usually done on an outpatient basis.

Gynaecologists have their own preferred ways of doing it. It has sometimes been used to reduce the size of large, embedded fibroids before myomectomy. After pretreatment with GnRH drugs for three months, the fibroids are drilled with the laser. This makes the fibroids less embedded, and thus easier to remove several weeks later by more conventional surgery.

But now myolysis is also being used as a complete treatment in its own right. Drugs are given beforehand for three months to shrink the fibroids. If they don't shrink, experience shows that myolysis will not work. If drugs are not used, there is also more likelihood of myolysis causing red degeneration in a fibroid.

A laparoscope is put into the abdomen, and the fibroid is then drilled either with a laser or a bipolar needle. The needle has an electric current passing between the two poles of the probe. The latest research suggests that it is better to use the needle because it causes less scarring than the laser.

Myolysis has been used on intramural fibroids up to 10 cm across. It takes about 30 minutes thoroughly to drill an 8-cm fibroid, according to one report. Myolysis is also used for fibroids in difficult positions – such as a cervical fibroid which is near the ureters – or for large fibroids which can't be tackled in any other way. One expert in myolysis says that the technique is best used on fibroids which are causing pressure problems. This specialist also says that myolysis may be the answer if you do not want a hysterectomy but have lots of fibroids, which would make a conventional myomectomy difficult. However myolysis could take too long if there are lots of fibroids.

Advantages of myolsis

Myolysis is simpler and quicker than laparoscopic myomectomy, because the fibroids do not have to be chopped up and removed. Benefits include a quick recovery time. There is little pain associated with myolysis, though you may have mild abdominal cramps for a few hours afterwards. You may well go home the same day, and be back to normal within a couple of days. Blood transfusions are rare with myolysis, and there are few post-operative infections and complications, according to research reports. Adhesions rarely form, particularly if the bipolar needle is used.

The evidence so far is that myolysis is an effective way of dealing with fibroids. In one study of 150 patients in which the laser was used, only one patient needed to have the procedure done a second time to reduce fibroid size. Drug therapy beforehand reduces fibroid size by between 30 to 50 per cent, and myolysis by another 30 to 50 per cent. Long-term follow-up suggests that the fibroids do not regrow.

Disadvantages of myolysis

Myolysis was originally developed as an alternative to myomectomy for women who wanted to have children. But it's unclear how much the procedure weakens the womb-wall, which might then rupture during pregnancy. Myolysis is therefore currently only recommended for women who don't want children, or who have completed their family. Some fibroids are also so hard that it's impossible to insert the probe. Finally, as with any surgical procedure, there's always the possibility that the abdomen may have to be opened up if there are complications.

Far more research still needs to be done into the advantages and disadvantages of myolysis. If you are interested in it, you must consult an expert in myolysis techniques.

The future

It may be possible eventually to block off the blood vessels leading to the fibroid. But this technique is at a very early stage, and it's unclear whether it's safe to use because it may cause clots elsewhere in the body.

Summary

- There are now various ways of doing a myomectomy. Each method has its advantages and disadvantages. Talk to your gynaecologist about what would be best for you, given your particular type of fibroids.
- If you are interested in having a myomectomy, but no mention is made of the procedure – or if the gynaecologist says it's only offered to women who want children – ask to see another specialist.
- Try to find out how experienced the gynaecologist is in myomectomy techniques.

- Ask about recovery time and what to expect after the procedure.
- GnRH drugs are used before most procedures, but the drugs may cause unpleasant side-effects.
- There is always a risk that keyhole surgery may turn into a conventional operation because of complications. A hysterectomy may occasionally be necessary if bleeding cannot be controlled.
- There is a one in four chance that fibroids could regrow after myomectomy, but if this happens they may remain symptomless, though they could cause problems again.
- Hysterectomy may be more difficult once you've had a myomectomy.

8

Hysterectomy

Hysterectomy – the removal of the womb – is one of the most commonly performed operations. Over 1,000 operations are carried out each week in this country, and it's estimated that about one in five women will have had the operation by the age of 65. One of the main reasons for a hysterectomy is fibroids.

Many gynaecologists still regard a hysterectomy as the best way to deal with troublesome fibroids, because it is a permanent solution: fibroids cannot regrow once the womb has been removed. With some exceptions, doctors tend to be particularly keen to do a hysterectomy if you are near to the menopause, rather than offering drug treatments or doing a myomectomy. As one gynaecologist put it: 'You don't know when the menopause is going to happen – it may not be as soon as you think. Women struggle on trying to cope with their symptoms but in the end they may need a hysterectomy.'

Elaine's story

Elaine, 53, had her fibroid diagnosed when she was in her mid-forties. She thinks her hormone-levels had started changing when she was about 43, as she'd started getting hot flushes. She's been waiting for the menopause ever since, and has suffered from erratic periods which can sometimes be very heavy, as well as back-pain. 'I keep thinking I'm at the menopause and this will be the end of my problems. But then I have another period.'

From the doctor's viewpoint, a hysterectomy is the obvious solution to fibroids which give rise to symptoms. However, some women are fearful of surgery or do not want to lose their womb.

Sarah's story

Sarah says: 'The gynaecologist wanted to take everything out – not only my womb but also my ovaries – because she was worried they might be cancerous. I think she also thought I wouldn't want to keep my womb because I was in my early fifties. But I didn't want another major operation, unless it really was necessary, because I'd had a lot of time off work for other health problems. I also wondered how the gynaecologist could know my ovaries were cancerous without taking a tissue sample from them. If I'd had everything out, I would have had to take HRT – but I'm worried about taking this because of the risk of developing breast cancer. I have a cousin who had everything removed, was put on to HRT and then developed breast cancer.'

Sandra's story

Sandra, 50, has managed for the past few years to avoid having a hysterectomy. 'I didn't want one because I wanted to have a child. But I'm also terrified of surgery, and just wanted to try and manage my heavy periods. I've now been told that I've got to have a hysterectomy because the fibroid is causing several problems. It presses on my bladder, and I have to go to the loo every hour and several times in the night. It's also uncomfortable making love. I'm going ahead with the operation – reluctantly.'

Louise's story

Louise, 41, says: 'I was adamant that I didn't want a hysterectomy when it was suggested in 1995. Far too many women are pushed into having one. I wanted to keep open my option to have children. But I also think it affects you psychologically if your womb is removed. I like having my womb. It makes me feel like a woman. I also like having my monthly period. I've had lots of problems with my periods at times, but when I have one I think everything is in working order. It makes me feel normal and I feel reassured. For me, it's part of my identity and a good monthly event.'

Jill's story

Others feel differently. Jill has suffered for years from fibroid symptoms and now, aged 50, would like to have a hysterectomy. But she has been told to hang on and see if her fibroid symptoms get better at the menopause.

Janet's story

Janet suffered from symptoms for several years, and was diagnosed as having fibroids when she was 38 years old. 'I had everything out and felt wonderful afterwards. I'd had such a rough time before with difficult periods, mood swings, tiredness and a lumpy stomach.

Love-making was also difficult, and we had to avoid deep penetration. Initially I had an argument with the gynaecologist who said I was too young to have a hysterectomy – but eventually it was agreed I could have one. I felt human afterwards, and found my moods were much better.'

Susan's story

Susan's periods became irregular and very heavy six years ago, when she was in her late thirties. She had a D&C, but then started getting a lot of period pain so she had an ultrasound scan which revealed a fibroid in the womb-lining. 'I coped for a time with drug treatment, but then I started getting periods every fortnight, as well as bleeding between periods. I saw another gynaecologist who examined me and said my womb was completely distorted. He advised me to have a hysterectomy.

'I had the operation a couple of months ago. My womb and ovaries were removed – apparently, apart from the fibroid, I had ovarian cysts as well as endometriosis. I was in hospital for seven days and suffered no real discomfort. Nine weeks later I'm back to normal, and I look and feel good. The operation was a great success and I wish I'd had it done all those years ago. I was so worried about having a hysterectomy – but now I don't know what all the fuss was about.'

There are various issues to consider if you are thinking about having a hysterectomy, or if your gynaecologist suggests one. Sometimes the operation is necessary if there's cancer in any of the pelvic organs, or if the womb has dropped down into the vagina – but it's estimated that only about one hysterectomy in ten is really necessary. As we've seen, there are other medical and surgical treatments – though you may have to fight for these. If you're unhappy about having a hysterectomy, take your time and check out the other options.

Don't let yourself be forced into having one. It's a question of weighing up the troublesomeness of your fibroids against the benefits and risks of surgery. Bear in mind that gynaecologists prefer some treatments to others. If your gynaecologist is adamant that you must have a hysterectomy, and if you don't want one, talk to your GP about the possibility of getting a second opinion from another gynaecologist, who may well have a different viewpoint.

Types of hysterectomy

There are various types of hysterectomy. You may not be presented with any choice about which procedure you have – for example, if the fibroid is cancerous. But depending on your medical condition, there may be a choice, for example, between a total hysterectomy, a vaginal hysterectomy or sub-total operation. As always, gynaecologists have procedures which they favour and so regularly perform. This means that they are skilled in this procedure – but not necessarily in the other methods. When you are discussing possible options, ask what experience they have in the various procedures.

Total abdominal hysterectomy

This is often used to remove large, bulky wombs containing fibroids. A cut is made just under the pubic hairline to remove the womb and neck of the womb – though a vertical incision may be made if the womb is very large.

The blood-vessels are clamped, and the Fallopian tubes and ovaries left in place. The womb, ovaries and pelvis are checked for signs of disease. The womb is then separated from the connective tissue surrounding it. A cut is made round the vagina where it meets the cervix, which is then pulled out and removed with the rest of the womb. The top of the vagina is then stitched. The abdominal incision is closed when all bleeding has stopped. The operation takes about an hour, depending on what needs doing.

You'll be in hospital for about seven days after this operation – and longer if there are complications. Full recovery varies, but can take about six to eight weeks. Some women say they find love-making less pleasurable because the cervix has been removed – this is discussed at the end of the chapter. You'll no longer need cervical smears, as the cervix has been removed.

Hysterectomy with removal of the ovaries

A hysterectomy with removal of the ovaries (total abdominal hysterectomy with bilateral salpingo-oophorectomy) involves not only removing the womb and cervix but also the ovaries and Fallopian tubes. Diseased ovaries clearly must be removed. The surgeon will also want to do this type of hysterectomy if the fibroid is cancerous, to prevent cancer spreading elsewhere in the pelvis.

But if you are near the menopause, quite a few gynaecologists are keen to remove healthy ovaries as a protection against ovarian cancer developing later on – particularly if you have a family history of ovarian cancer.

If both your ovaries are removed before the menopause, you will have a surgical menopause and experience menopausal symptoms straightaway. These include hot flushes, night sweats, insomnia, mood swings, poor memory and concentration, vaginal dryness, depression and sometimes loss of sex-drive. But symptoms can be more severe after a surgical menopause because of the sudden withdrawal of oestrogen. In a non-surgical menopause, oestrogen-levels decline gradually over a number of years. Without the same level of oestrogen in the body, women also become more vulnerable to long-term problems such as osteoporosis (the bone-thinning disease) and heart disease.

HRT (hormone replacement therapy) is given after this operation to relieve short-term symptoms and protect women against long-term problems.

Susan's story

Susan starting taking HRT after her operation. So far she's had no side-effects from the HRT, and feels much better than she did before she had the operation.

Worries about removing the ovaries

Doctors often argue that removal of the ovaries is not a problem, because HRT can be taken. But HRT may be insufficient to provide relief from symptoms which can be particularly severe after a surgical menopause. Some gynaecologists also claim that bone-thinning is greater after a menopause brought about by surgery. There are also worries and conflicting reports about whether or not HRT, taken long term, may slightly increase the risk of breast cancer. One study suggests that the risk might increase after five years, and another after ten years. However, the latest study found no increased risk after 15 years – though this by no means puts an end to this debate.

Another recent study reports a possible link between HRT and blood-clots. Some women are also not able to take HRT for various health reasons, and others suffer side-effects, such as mood swings and headaches. There is also research suggesting that some women can become addicted to HRT and may need increasing amounts of it to gain any relief from symptoms. Advocates of HRT, however, argue that its side-effects can be remedied by changing to a different product, as there is a large range of HRT preparations. They claim that the solution is to find the type of HRT which suits you.

It's best to talk through any concerns you have with your gynaecologist when mention is first made of hysterectomy. If you do not want your ovaries removed, make sure that the surgeon who is doing your operation knows your wishes. As discussed in Chapter 5, you can also make alterations to the consent form. But the best bet is to let the surgeon know how you feel. It's sensible to try to prevent problems occurring, rather than having to deal with the consequences later on.

Sub-total hysterectomy

In this operation, only the womb is removed. This type of hysterectomy is little-used at the moment. According to one survey, less than 1 per cent of women have a sub-total hysterectomy.

Surgeons have been unhappy about leaving the neck of the womb in place because of the risk of cervical cancer developing. One specialist explained that there were various reasons for this: it is, for example, harder to treat cervical cancer after a sub-total hysterectomy because it is more difficult surgically to remove the cervix. Another expert was deeply opposed to this type of hysterectomy. From his viewpoint, the cervix was a source of potential problems: it could become cancerous, or get infected and cause discharges. Some women are worried about having the cervix removed because they fear their sex-life may suffer, but he said there was no independent evidence that removal of the cervix affected sexual pleasure.

But the sub-total hysterectomy may come back into fashion, despite opposition to it. Another specialist was certainly prepared to perform this operation in what he described as 'the right circumstances'. He pointed out that it may be safe to leave your cervix in place if, for example, you are 50 and have always had normal smear results. But if you have had abnormal results, he would advise removal of the neck of the womb.

Apart from the question about the cervix and sexual pleasure, there are other advantages to the sub-total hysterectomy. It's an easier operation than the total abdominal hysterectomy, and the risk of infection is reduced because the vagina is not opened up. There's also less risk of damage to the bladder. Hospital stay is shorter, and recovery quicker – and you will probably feel less traumatized by this procedure. However, you still need to keep having cervical smears. If you want to keep your cervix, discuss the possibility of having this type of hysterectomy with your gynaecologist. If there is no good reason why you shouldn't have it done, but the gynaecologist refuses to do a sub-total hysterectomy, try to see another specialist.

Vaginal hysterectomy

A vaginal hysterectomy is similar to a total abdominal hysterectomy – but the womb and cervix are removed through the vagina. The advantage of this operation is that recovery time is quicker – about five weeks as opposed to two months – because there is no abdominal incision. The stay in hospital is about half that for an abdominal operation. In skilled hands, complications are rare with this procedure – though there is always the possibility of infection and possible damage to the bladder and ureters. The operation takes about an hour.

It may not be possible to have this type of hysterectomy if your womb is very bulky as a result of having fibroids. But it should be possible to use this procedure for a womb up to the size of a 10–12-week pregnancy – which covers a large number of cases, according to one expert. However, one specialist has reported removing more bulky wombs – up to the size of a 20-week pregnancy – by the vaginal route. GnRH drugs are given for several months beforehand to shrink the womb. However, removing large wombs vaginally may be risky, and may lead to more complications unless the gynaecologist is an expert.

There are other reasons why it may not be possible to have this operation. Diseased ovaries cannot be removed by vaginal hysterectomy. Nor can the womb be removed through the vagina if it is stuck in the abdomen as a result of scarring due to previous surgery. So, for instance, if you've had an abdominal myomectomy in the past, you may find that your gynaecologist is reluctant to do a vaginal hysterectomy.

Some gynaecologists are very keen on this procedure because they say it is less invasive. However, it cannot always be done because of the problems just outlined. According to a 1992 study, only about four per cent of hysterectomies were performed vaginally.

Laparoscopically assisted vaginal hysterectomy

This procedure is available in a few centres but – like laparoscopic myomectomy – it takes longer to perform than the conventional abdominal operation. According to one expert, it's a way of converting an abdominal hysterectomy into a vaginal hysterectomy, with all its benefits. But the procedure still needs a lot more evaluation.

The abdomen is inflated with gas and the laparoscope inserted into the abdomen just underneath the navel. Surgical instruments are inserted through two other tiny incisions. The womb is cut free from surrounding tissue and then removed through the vagina, as in vaginal hysterectomy.

This method can be used if your womb is glued to the abdomen with scar-tissue, as this can be cut away. The ovaries can also be removed if necessary. Recovery time is much quicker than after a conventional abdominal hysterectomy – about three weeks, as opposed to two to three months – because the abdomen is punctured rather than cut. But the operation takes a long time – perhaps three hours as compared to one hour. The complication rate can also be high unless the gynaecologist is expert in doing keyhole surgery.

Wertheim's hysterectomy

Wertheim's hysterectomy – also known as a radical hysterectomy – is carried out when there's cancer in the cervix. It consists of the removal of the womb, both ovaries and Fallopian tubes, the cervix and the top part of the vagina, the lymph glands, as well as the ligaments that support the womb, and fatty tissue in the pelvis.

Before and after the operation

It's important to prepare for a major operation as outlined in Chapter 7. There is less risk of needing a blood transfusion during a hysterectomy than in an abdominal myomectomy. But it may still be worth talking to your gynaecologist about whether to save some of your own blood beforehand.

To prepare for a hysterectomy:

- It's important to be as fit as possible for the operation.
- If you are going to have a vaginal hysterectomy, it's particularly important to do pelvic-floor exercises beforehand to make sure the pelvic-floor muscles are in good shape.

- If you're overweight, lose excess pounds: Elaine has actually been told she can't have a hysterectomy except in an emergency because she is so overweight.
- Eat a well-balanced diet.
- If you smoke, try to give up before surgery.
- Stop taking the combined contraceptive Pill several weeks before the operation.

After the operation, you will have an intravenous drip in a vein in your arm, to replace fluids lost during the operation. You may also have a catheter inserted into your bladder to drain away urine. The tube will be removed to see if you can pass urine. It's important that you pass urine within 12 hours after the operation, to prevent the bladder from getting enlarged. About one woman in ten is unable to do this. If this is the case, the catheter is put back in and removed a couple of days later. You may also have a drainage tube in the abdomen to remove blood. You'll also have some light vaginal bleeding after the operation, which may go on for a few weeks. Use pads rather than tampons. Let medical staff know if bleeding becomes heavy, as this may be a sign of internal bleeding. A smelly discharge could be a sign of infection.

It's normal to have some pain. Some women find this lasts for a day or so; others may need painkilling injections for several days. Expect to feel tired. You may also feel a bit depressed for a couple of days or so. There is no feeling of emptiness inside your abdomen after the womb is removed, as other organs move to fill the space left by the womb. Your vagina is the same size as before – unless you had the Wertheim's hysterectomy.

As soon as possible after the operation, you should start doing gentle movements to get your circulation moving, to prevent clots forming in the deep veins in the body. After the anaesthetic it's important to get your lungs moving. Regular, deep breathing will help do this. (Various exercises for movement and breathing were described in Chapter 7.)

Pelvic-floor exercises (described in Chapter 10) are important because they strengthen the pelvic floor and improve muscle-tone. They will help ease discomfort and improve bladder-control, as well as keeping your vagina healthy and preventing future incontinence problems. The exercises will also guard against prolapse of any of the pelvic organs. A physiotherapist should show you how to do these, as well as other exercises which will help relieve back-ache and wind.

When you go home – the timing will depend on which procedure you've had – you'll need to rest, and take time to get back to normal. Don't do anything which involves heavy lifting for the first 12 weeks, as tissue and muscles need time to heal and get back to normal. If you do lift anything, bend your knees, pull in your stomach and pelvic-floor muscles, and keep your back straight. The gynaecologist will check you about six weeks after the operation to make sure that everything has healed properly.

You shouldn't start doing any competitive sports until about three months afterwards. Swimming may be possible after your six-week check-up. Gentle walking is good: try ten minutes each day initially, gradually increasing this as you become stronger. After your six-week check-up you should be able to make love again – before then you may have some bleeding. If your ovaries remain in place, you'll keep having a monthly cycle – but obviously you will no longer have periods, as the womb has been removed.

Points to consider

Hysterectomy is a major operation. It's therefore important to weigh up various points in order to decide whether it's right for you (though in a few cases there may be no option – if, for example, there is cancer anywhere in the pelvis). Many women are very satisfied with their hysterectomy – I spoke to women who wished they had not waited so long before having the operation. But you should consider the following points.

- As discussed in Chapter 7, a hysterectomy may be more difficult to do if you have previously had a myomectomy.
- Surgery always carries risks. There is always the risk of death (though death-rates are low for hysterectomy at around one per thousand). After the operation, various problems can occur – though these are usually of a minor nature. But more serious complications can occur; however, risks will be minimized if an experienced surgeon does the operation.
- According to one estimate, one in four women may suffer from various complications afterwards. These include wound infection, bladder or bowel damage, chest infections and blood-clots. Hae-morrhages can also occur during or after the operation.
- An important longer-term problem may be urinary incontinence or

the need to urinate frequently. The bladder is moved around a lot during a hysterectomy, and its nerve or blood-supply may be affected, causing pain and various symptoms. Bladder function can be permanently affected.

- If love-making is an important part of your life, it's important to consider the possible effects of a hysterectomy. If, before the operation, you have experienced lots of discomfort during sex, then your sex-life may be much better after a hysterectomy. But there doesn't seem to have been much research into the effects of the various types of hysterectomy on a woman's sexual enjoyment. Yet this is sometimes a very important issue. Some women reach orgasm as the penis thrusts against the cervix: obviously this is no longer possible when the cervix has been removed. Some studies show that the quality of orgasm is less satisfactory after a hysterectomy, and that some women find it more difficult to have an orgasm.

- Your love-life may also be affected if you are pre-menopausal and have your ovaries removed – which will give you a surgical menopause. As a result of the sudden decline in oestrogen in your body, you may experience acute menopausal symptoms. You may find that your sex-drive is much lower, and that your vagina is dry. As discussed earlier in the chapter, HRT is used to treat menopausal symptoms when the ovaries are removed – but you may still experience problems.

- If you have a hysterectomy, you may have an earlier menopause – even if your ovaries remain. When the womb is removed, the blood-supply to the ovaries may be affected – which can bring about a menopause perhaps one to two years earlier than would have occurred without the operation. This means an increased risk of osteoporosis and heart problems – though HRT can provide some protection against these longer-term problems. Some doctors do a blood-test to check hormone-levels to try and assess whether the menopause is occurring earlier, so that HRT can be prescribed.

Summary

Some women are absolutely clear that they want a hysterectomy – but others are worried about having major surgery, or may not want to lose what they see as a vital part of themselves. Don't rush into it. It's easy to feel you are losing control and being pushed into an operation you are not sure you want – but remember, the decision is yours. Take your time: read about the various types of hysterectomy; talk to women who have been through it. Some women say their lives have taken a turn for the worse after the operation – but many others say the opposite. Talk to your gynaecologist about the various options, and which would be best for you.

9

Non-conventional treatments

Is it worth trying out non-conventional treatments (often referred to as complementary or alternative therapies) if you have symptom-causing fibroids? Complementary therapies are becoming popular, and it's claimed they can be effective for a range of conditions – but most of the women I spoke to had not tried them. Sally's attitude was typical.

Sally's story

'I'm very busy', Sally said. 'I'm a parent and have a very demanding job, and it's cheaper and simpler for me to try the conventional route. If the pills don't work I might consider trying acupuncture for my period problems.'

Laura's story

Laura, however, has tried other approaches – such as aromatherapy, reflexology and spiritual healing – because she has still not been able to have a successful pregnancy, despite having had various drug and surgical treatments.

Complementary therapies tend to be considered when all else has failed – though some people are committed from the outset to using these approaches instead of conventional ones. If your fibroids are causing pressure symptoms, the fibroids will probably need to be surgically removed. But there is a place for complementary therapies in the treatment of period problems caused by fibroids. They can also be used alongside conventional treatments, to improve health generally.

There are a huge number of non-conventional therapies – around 700 on offer – and this can pose problems if you are trying to decide which one is right for you. One researcher has divided therapies into four groups (though there are other ways of trying to distinguish between therapies). One group contains therapies such as homeopathy and herbalism which are described as complete systems of healing. The second group, which includes therapies such as hair analysis and iridology, are seen to be mainly concerned with diagnosis. The third group is described as therapeutic approaches, such as massage and reflexology. The fourth group, which includes yoga and relaxation techniques, is defined as self-care approaches. In this chapter, we shall look at some of the therapies in the first group – as well as others which may be of particular use. Some of the therapies in the last two groups are considered in Chapter 10.

Non-conventional approaches have one important point in common: they stress the importance of using a holistic approach to health. They look at the health of both mind and body, and try to get to the root of the problem rather than just treating symptoms. They often talk about being in balance and at ease with yourself. Their aim is to stimulate the body's own powers of healing. Don't expect an overnight cure if you try a complementary therapy. Treatment may continue over a period of weeks, if not months, and possibly for a year while the body is rebalanced.

These non-conventional therapies have increasingly become accepted as part of the NHS. Some 'conventional' doctors also use homeopathic or other complementary therapy skills, and many GPs are happy to refer patients to non-conventional therapists.

There are a few points to consider before looking at specific therapies. Anecdotal reports describe how some therapies have helped women with fibroids. However, there are few if any large, well-designed research studies that show whether any of the therapies are effective in the treatment of fibroid symptoms. The studies that do exist tend to be case reports which give information about one patient's treatment and the outcome.

But these studies are meaningless in statistical terms. Random controlled trials, used to evaluate conventional treatments, are thought to be the best way of trying to judge the effectiveness of particular treatments. Patients are allocated at random to two different groups (the patients themselves not knowing which group they are in): one group is given a sham treatment (called a placebo), and the other the real treatment. The results are then compared and evaluated. It's often argued that non-conventional therapies should be subjected to the same evaluation. But therapists often argue that non-conventional therapies can't be analysed in this way, because treatments are tailor-made for each individual. It's also argued that you can't give a dummy treatment in some of the therapies. In acupuncture, for instance, how do you give a dummy needle? Supporters of complementary therapies also rightly point out that many conventional treatments have not been properly evaluated.

Some doctors dismiss complementary therapies as of unproven value. One doctor was keen to point out that any benefit felt by patients was due to the large amount of time and attention given to them, rather than to the actual therapy itself. This whole area is complex, and open to much debate – but you should be aware of it if you want to use any of these approaches. The more you expect from complementary therapies, the more important this issue becomes. Conventional treatments are not exempt from questions about whether or not they work, and the same questions should be asked about complementary therapies. As with conventional treatment it's best if possible to see a therapist who is interested and experienced in treating fibroid problems. Ask your doctor whether you can see a therapist under the NHS. If not, you will have to pay for treatment. If this is the case, find out what treatment sessions cost and how many you're likely to need.

One of the attractions of complementary therapies is that they are usually seen as totally safe and free of side-effects – unlike conventional treatments. But, as with any treatment, there can be problems in untrained hands. So it's important that you see a registered practitioner – and before you agree to any treatment, ask about possible side-effects, and the risks of any proposed treatment.

With some of the therapies – notably homeopathy and acupuncture – there is another point to consider. Do you want to see a doctor who has acquired these skills in addition to conventional medical skills, or do you want to see a lay person who has trained as a therapist? Lay practitioners tend to argue that GPs who become acupuncturists or homeopaths have undergone a less rigorous training, and so may be less effective therapists. Conversely, GPs tend to argue that lay practitioners don't have enough training in general medicine, and so could make important mistakes.

Specific therapies

I have looked at various research papers and talked to some therapists. From my research I have concluded that the most useful therapies for fibroids are probably homeopathy and herbalism. Traditional Chinese medicine and acupuncture are reputed to be useful – though I was able to find out less about these approaches. The other therapies I've listed also have a part to play – but perhaps more in a supporting role. It's best if you can get your doctor and therapist to work together in helping you. In this way you get the best of both worlds. For example, your doctor can organize ultrasound scans to check what's happening to your fibroids and blood-tests to check for anaemia, if you are having homeopathy.

Homeopathy

Homeopathy is based on the idea that like may be cured by like. A substance that causes symptoms in a healthy person can cure those symptoms in an ill person. Symptoms are seen as the body's attempt to overcome disease. Instead of suppressing symptoms, the idea is to stimulate them as part of the healing process. Homeopathy uses extremely dilute doses of plant, animal and mineral substances to boost the body's immune system. Homeopathic remedies are considered to be completely safe with no side-effects, as well as being non-addictive because the substances are so weak.

The choice of remedy depends more on your individual reaction to illness, mentally and emotionally, than on the signs and symptoms characteristic of the disease – according to the British Homeopathic Association. The initial consultation with a homeopath is lengthy. You are asked many details about your medical history and personality.

Homeopathy is often described as one of the complementary therapies which is particularly useful for women's health problems. And homeopathy can help fibroid problems, according to a 1992 article in the *British Homeopathic Journal*. Eighty-four patients with troublesome fibroids were treated only with homeopathy, and monitored with ultrasound scans and pelvic examination over one to three years. According to the researchers, the results show that homeopathy on its own is an effective method for treating fibroids. They claim that it is possible to stop fibroids growing, and even to reduce their size, as well as treating pain and abnormal bleeding, with homeopathic remedies.

This study can undoubtedly be criticized on a number of points – not least of which is that this was not a random controlled trial. But though there may be various problems with it (as there are with most research trials), it is at least an attempt to evaluate the effectiveness of homeopathy for fibroids.

I spoke to a couple of doctors who have also trained as homeopaths. One said that homeopathy is an effective treatment because it helps the body heal itself, whereas other approaches relieve symptoms but do not cure the underlying problem. In other words, homeopathy stimulates the body's capacity for self-healing. He explained that homeopathy can be used in two ways:

1 By treating a specific problem on a short-term basis – for instance, Secale is used for heavy bleeding, or Aconite for sudden, torrential flooding.
2 Homeopathy can be used for chronic problems by preparing a tailor-made constitutional remedy for each person's specific emotional and physical make-up.

However, he thought that the remedies would not be able to shrink large fibroids because, by this stage, the disease would have progressed too far.

The other doctor agreed that homeopathy can help with heavy periods, but specifically said that there is not yet enough evidence to suggest that homeopathic remedies can shrink fibroids. She explained that homeopathy can be used as a first-line treatment for heavy bleeding for three to six months. In her experience, the remedies are more effective at stopping heavy bleeding than conventional drug treatments. She also advised that, during homeopathic treatment, fibroids should be monitored with ultrasound scans, and that blood-tests be done to check for anaemia. This approach combines the benefits of conventional and non-conventional medicine.

Herbalism

Herbs have been used for thousands of years for health problems and many modern drugs are derived from plants.

Judy's story

Judy, 44, decided to try herbalism to see if it could help her symptoms. 'The gynaecologist told me last year that I had a fibroid the size of a grapefruit, and that I was anaemic because of it. We

105

decided to monitor the fibroid and review the situation in a few months – though he really wanted me to have a hysterectomy. But as far as I was concerned, I'd had no problems apart from the fact that my periods were a bit heavier. I wasn't keen on surgery. The fibroid hasn't got any bigger, but I decided to see a herbalist recently because I was feeling tired. She's put me on medicine to improve my circulation and reduce my bleeding. I expect to have herbal treatment for about a year. It's very early days, but I already feel less tired.'

Sandy's story

Sandy saw a herbalist ten years ago when she was 29. 'I wanted to get pregnant and was told I had this large fibroid. I went away and did some research, and decided to consult a herbalist. He said it would take some years to break down the fibroid with herbal treatment and that it would be best, if I wanted to get pregnant, to have a myomectomy. So I decided to have the operation – but for a couple of months beforehand, the herbalist gave me a mixture of herbs to take three times a day. When I had the operation the consultant was pleasantly surprised that the fibroid hadn't got any bigger, and that no smaller ones had appeared.'

Diana's story

Diana, 43, is using herbs to self-treat her fibroids. 'When I was pregnant at the age of 30, a fibroid was discovered during a routine scan, but it didn't cause any problems. However, last year my period was late and my abdomen became rather swollen, so I thought I might be pregnant. I had an abdominal scan and fibroids were diagnosed. The doctor told me that my womb was the size of a 16-week pregnancy, and that I should have a hysterectomy. But I really don't want this unless it's absolutely necessary. My womb is part of my sexuality, and I get a lot of pleasure from it during orgasm so I don't want it removed.

'I can feel the fibroid, and it seems to vary in size during my cycle. But otherwise I haven't got any other symptoms and I have no other pelvic conditions. Earlier this year I decided to use the herbs for fibroids described in Rina Nissim's book, *Natural Healing in Gynecology*, to see if the fibroids would get smaller. My breasts are now less swollen before my period, and the period itself is less heavy. I only have a heavy flow on one day, whereas before I bled heavily for two to three days. My periods are about the same length, but my cycle is slightly shorter and more regular than previously. I'm also trying to cut out fat from my diet. But so far my womb still seems pretty bulky, and I'm waiting to see if it gets smaller.'

For another woman, symptom relief is all that matters: in the *Women's Health* leaflet on fibroids, she explains that since she started herbal treatment her periods have become less troublesome. But she feels that the fibroids are still the same size – that of a 16-week pregnancy. However, she says a hysterectomy is unnecessary because she feels fit and well.

I spoke to a couple of herbalists, members of the National Institute of Medical Herbalists, set up in 1864. They said that herbalism can help fibroid problems – and they also emphasized that it's important for the herbalist and doctor to co-operate with each other. In their view, poor circulation in the pelvis may in some way contribute to fibroid problems. The following points emerged.

- Herbalists treat the individual, and aim to put the body back in balance.
- A herbalist would first deal with any immediate problems (such as heavy bleeding) and then use herbs to try and shrink the fibroids – apparently some fibroids do get smaller.
- Herbalists give dietary guidance. You are likely to get advice about following a low-oestrogen diet – for example, cutting down on dairy products and meat, and eating more fish, whole grains, seeds and pulses. A herbalist might prescribe a cleansing diet to help remove poisons from the body.
- Herbs may be given to improve circulation as well as to correct hormonal imbalance. The herb *vitex agnus castus*, commonly known as chaste berry or monk's pepper, is one of the most important herbs used to regulate female hormone problems, according to an article in the 1994 *European Journal of Herbal Medicine*. Fibroids are one of the conditions for which it is used.
- Herbs can be given to treat anaemia.
- Sitz baths may be recommended, to get energy moving in the pelvis. This involves sitting in a bath of cold water for a couple of minutes,

then in hot water for a couple of minutes – and repeating this procedure several times.

• Some herbs can be harmful, so it's important not to self-treat but to see a qualified herbalist.

Acupuncture

Chinese medicine has a different view of illness from Western medicine. Traditional acupuncture aims to treat the whole person, and thinks that illness is caused by blockages of energy in invisible channels in the body. Acupuncture is used for all sorts of health problems, including period problems. Members of the British Acupuncture Council are not usually doctors, but will have been through a two- to four-year training to become qualified. Traditional acupuncturists don't talk about fibroids as such, but see the growths as a symptom of a broader imbalance in the body. They claim that they can treat fibroid problems successfully.

If you see a traditional acupuncturist, expect to be asked lots of questions about your medical history, your family and your symptoms. The questions could take an hour or so. The acupuncturist will want to know about your energy levels, and will ask you about what you like to eat, your reactions to heat or cold and how you sleep. The practitioner will feel for various pulses in your wrist, and will probably look at your tongue. You'll feel a mild pin-prick and perhaps a twinge as needles are placed a little under the skin at appropriate points on the network of invisible channels. The needles may be gently manipulated, or just left in place for 15 minutes or so, and then removed. You may only need one or two sessions over a couple of weeks – but treatment can sometimes last several months.

The British Acupuncture Society, whose members are doctors, emphasized that, though acupuncture can be used to treat symptoms of pain and general discomfort in the abdomen, it could not shrink fibroids.

Chinese herbal medicine

Herbs are also used extensively in Chinese medicine. A herbal remedy, *Keishi-bukuryo-gan*, was used in one study of 110 patients with fibroids. The researchers claimed that the remedy reduced heavy bleeding in 90 per cent of women, and that the fibroids shrank in 60 per cent of women. If you want to try Chinese herbal medicine, make sure you see a doctor properly qualified in using traditional Chinese medicine. The herbs can be dangerous in unskilled hands.

Chiropractic

Chiropractors use their hands to manipulate joints and muscles, particularly those in the spine. I decided to speak to a practitioner because I'd come across a paper which referred to the use of a treatment, called total mesenteric apron, for fibroid problems in two women.

The chiropractor explained that the womb and ovaries may not work efficiently if the area of the back which controls them isn't working properly. She said that problems such as clotting, painful periods and heavy bleeding can be treated successfully by working on this part of the back. But she stressed that it's always important to see a doctor first to get a proper diagnosis. A chiropractor would aim to get everything functioning properly again. Dietary changes may also be recommended. If you're fairly inactive, the therapist may suggest exercises to keep the back mobile and to exercise the pelvic-floor muscles. Again, there are no set treatments for fibroid problems, as treatment is tailored to the individual. If you want to try this approach, ask to see a chiropractor who has specialized in this treatment.

Osteopathy

Osteopathy seems to offer a similar approach. Osteopaths will shortly be registered by law, so you have the same protection as when you visit a doctor or a dentist. Osteopaths also work with their hands to diagnose and treat problems. I spoke to an osteopath who explained that the techniques can be used to help prevent problems occurring, and can be used in conjunction with conventional medical treatment. The therapist aims to restore the proper nerve-supply from the lower back to the womb – though fibroids are probably more to do with oestrogen imbalance, the therapist said. Again, treatment would vary and is tailor-made, and you would be advised to get a proper medical diagnosis first. It's worth considering osteopathy for fibroid problems if you have low back-pain or if you've unsuccessfully tried conventional methods. Again, try to make sure you see an osteopath who is experienced in treating fibroid problems.

Nutritional therapy

Nutritional therapy is increasingly fashionable at the moment. According to the Society for the Promotion of Nutritional Therapy, which was established in 1991, nutritional therapy is more than just healthy eating. It is a natural health-care system which uses various diets, mineral, vitamin and sometimes herbal products, to help the body work more efficiently and heal itself. Specialist practitioners use diagnostic diets and biochemical tests to identify the root-cause of a patient's symptoms.

It's likely you will be told that your fibroids are related to liver problems, and that you have some sort of hormone imbalance. According to this view, fibroids are the result of oestrogen-overload in the body, caused by the liver not breaking oestrogens down properly into a less active type of oestrogen. It's unclear why this should happen. The liver may not have been working properly in the first place, or may have had too many demands placed on it. The aim is to make the liver work more effectively so that it can do its job properly. It's important to see a qualified nutritional therapist if you want to explore whether this approach can help. Treatment may take some months before you experience the benefits.

Summary

- Always make sure you have a proper medical diagnosis before seeing a complementary therapist. Conventional medicine is best for diagnosis – not only to confirm that you have a fibroid, but also to check whether you have other co-existing pelvic conditions.
- Ideally it's best if your doctor and therapist can work together on your behalf.
- Make sure you see a qualified therapist and one who specializes in women's health – and if possible, who has a particular interest in fibroid problems. Ask if you can be referred to a therapist on the NHS – paying for complementary therapy privately can be very

expensive. Ask what's involved and how many treatment sessions you will need.

10
Living with fibroids

There are various things you can do to look after yourself if you have symptom-causing fibroids. Doing something to help yourself will also make you feel more in control of your life, which in itself is a good thing. Louise, who has had fibroids for many years, says that diet, rest and exercise have helped reduce the severity of her symptoms. Towards the end of the chapter, we look at the options available if you are worried about taking HRT, and also touch on the question of whether it's advisable to use the contraceptive Pill for birth control.

Anaemia

One of the most important things you can do is to prevent yourself from getting anaemic. If you suffer from heavy periods, it's important to make sure you're not suffering from iron-deficiency anaemia. Several women I spoke to suffered from this problem.

The sorts of symptoms to look out for include headaches, tiredness, weakness, lethargy, heart palpitations (a sensation of having a rapid and unusually forceful heartbeat), possible pallor in the creases of the skin, the lining of the mouth and the inside of the eyelids, and brittle nails. Not only does anaemia make you feel exhausted and ill – but also, if you suddenly need an operation, it may require you to have a blood transfusion beforehand. Anaemia can also affect you in other ways: your ability to concentrate may be reduced and you may feel apathetic. Your body's ability to protect itself from infection can also be impaired.

As discussed in Chapter 3, the oxygen-carrying capacity of the blood falls when levels of haemoglobin (the oxygen-carrying pigment) fall below normal. Iron-deficiency anaemia develops if insufficient iron is available in the bone-marrow, where haemoglobin is made and packaged into red blood-cells. Iron-deficiency anaemia occurs when iron-loss persistently exceeds iron gained from the diet.

This type of anaemia occurs for three main reasons:

1 through blood-loss;

2 because of poor absorption of iron from the diet;
3 a lack of iron in the diet.

So if you're having heavy, prolonged periods, you could be losing too much iron. For example, if your blood-loss is 118 ml per period (which is heavy) your daily iron-loss is about 1.9 mg over a 28-day cycle – as compared to an average daily loss of 0.7 mg for women with normal monthly blood-loss.

Not all women with heavy periods are anaemic, so it's important to have blood-tests to check haemoglobin-levels and iron stores in the body. If you simply assume you are lacking iron and take supplements accordingly, you could be accumulating excess iron in the body, which is harmful. Some women also have a genetic condition called haemochromatosis, which means they have excess iron in their bodies. Haemochromatosis sufferers should certainly not take iron supplements. It used to be thought that women couldn't develop symptoms of this disease before the menopause because of losing blood each month – but it's now known that iron-overload can sometimes develop before the menopause.

If you are diagnosed as being anaemic, make sure you ask your doctor about how to treat anaemia and then how to prevent it. I spoke to several women who said they weren't given any information about what supplements to take, though their doctor had confirmed they were anaemic. There are a various ways you can take iron – for instance, in tablet form, as capsules, or as syrups or elixirs in which iron-salts are dissolved in a mixture of alcohol and water. Always follow instructions about how to take the preparation. Syrups or elixirs should be sucked through a straw to try and prevent staining of the teeth. If supplements don't work, your doctor may give you an iron injection. A common way of doing this is to give several injections of iron into muscle over several days.

Iron preparations can cause side-effects, such as stomach upset, abdominal pain, nausea, vomiting, diarrhoea, constipation and black stools. If this happens ask your doctor or the pharmacist about changing to a product which suits you better.

Once your haemoglobin-levels are back to normal – within the range 11.5–16 g per 100 ml of blood – and you have sufficient iron stores, make sure you don't get anaemic again. Over-the-counter low-dosage iron products are available, designed to prevent anaemia. They are usually taken once a day. Get advice from your doctor and pharmacist about which products are most suitable for you.

But the best way to make sure you get enough iron is through your diet. Certain foods are rich in iron – for example liver, kidneys and offal in general, black treacle and dried fruit, red wine and dark chocolate. Experts advise eating a healthy, nutritious diet, with meals planned around certain foods, rather than planned around the iron-content of food portions.

Most of the iron in our diet is called non-haem iron, and comes from plant products (fruit and vegetables) and sometimes animal products. Haem iron is only found in animal products, and is much more easily absorbed than non-haem iron. If you are a vegetarian you need to be particularly careful that you get sufficient iron.

Try to ensure that you have a mixture of protein-rich foods, cereals, fruit and vegetables. Plenty of vitamin C will improve the absorption of iron from non-haem sources. Tannin (found in tea) can interfere with the body's absorption of iron: try not to drink tea or coffee immediately before or after a meal. Make sure you eat regularly throughout the day, so have breakfast, lunch and supper.

Sanitary protection

Dealing with bouts of heavy bleeding can be very distressing. It's worth experimenting with different types of sanitary protection to see if this can help you cope better – for example, using a tampon with a pad, and using extra-absorbent night-time protection.

Susan's story

Susan just about managed during the half-day or so when she had very heavy flooding. 'I used a super-plus tampon, together with a large sanitary towel – but I used to have to change my sanitary protection every 20 minutes or so when the bleeding was very heavy.'

Some women find they can also cope better by talking about the problem to their doctor, rather than suffering in silence. Talking about the problem to supportive women friends may also prove useful. If you're having very heavy periods, it's also important to remember that your periods may lighten again after some months – though of course it's impossible to know in advance when this is going to happen.

Diet

Louise's story

> Over ten years ago, Louise changed her diet after having her first myomectomy, aged 29. 'I cut out meat and dairy products, and started eating fish, whole grains, plenty of vegetables and seaweed. For ten years I wasn't troubled by fibroids, which I think is probably due in part to these dietary changes.'

The principle of a low-fat, healthy diet, with plenty of fresh fruit and vegetables, is one with which many of us are now familiar. It is accepted that what you eat can have significant implications for your health generally. But some people think that the right diet can rectify excessive oestrogen-levels in the body, and balance the female hormones. Since high oestrogen-levels are linked to fibroid growth, it is certainly worth thinking seriously about whether you can make changes to your diet so that, not only do you eat for general health, but also for female-hormone health.

As explained in Chapter 9, nutritional therapists and herbalists can discuss diet in more detail. Nutritional therapists can also advise about whether or not you need to take certain mineral and vitamin supplements, in addition to making dietary changes, and how to do so safely. There is a debate about whether you can get enough nutrients from food alone. Some therapists argue that you may need high doses of additional supplements to rectify vitamin and mineral deficiencies. They argue that at least half the UK population does not get enough nutrients each day from their diet to prevent deficiency problems.

You may be tempted to self-treat yourself with various supplements. Dietary supplements are often thought of as more natural, and so safer, than conventional medicines. However, this is not always so. High doses of vitamins and minerals may upset the body's delicate balance and cause various problems. For instance, high doses of vitamin B6 may harm nerve-function, and large doses of vitamin A can be poisonous. Large doses of zinc can cause anaemia. To get the best advice, and to make sure that you do yourself no harm, consult a nutritional therapist (as discussed in Chapter 9). For more conventional dietary advice, consult a dietician who can advise about healthy eating generally, but who is likely to say that there is no need for dietary supplements.

Useful foods

In general terms, it's important to have a varied diet. But certain foods may be particularly helpful, as explained in the following notes. You can help yourself by trying to make sure that you eat these foods regularly – but don't eat excessive amounts of any one food, as this might also cause problems. The following points are worth noting.

- In one study, vitamin A (also called retinol) levels were reduced in women who had heavy bleeding and flooding. After using vitamin A supplements, bleeding-patterns returned to normal. Vitamin A is necessary for the growth and maintenance of healthy skin and eyes, as well as for an effective immune system. Try to make sure you get plenty of vitamin A. Good sources include liver, herrings, sardines, eggs and carrots.
- The group of B vitamins are also thought to be important in regulating oestrogen-level, as well as reducing periods pains and cramps. The B vitamins are found particularly in whole grains, beans, peas, liver, nuts, bananas and avocado pears.
- Vitamin E is also important for female health. Good sources are wheatgerm (which can be sprinkled on cereal), walnuts, soybean oil and avocados.
- A high-fibre diet is also thought to help reduce oestrogen-levels in the body.
- Whole grains are a good source of magnesium, which helps ease period cramps.
- Vegetables are high in calcium, magnesium and potassium, and so also help reduce period cramps. Eat plenty of spinach, broccoli and potatoes – as well as seaweed, now increasingly available in shops.
- Essential fatty acids are important for hormone health, and can also ease period pain by encouraging muscle relaxation. Good sources include evening primrose oil, wheatgerm, linseed, sesame and sunflower seeds, unsalted nuts and fish such as salmon, mackerel and trout.

116

Plant oestrogens

Angela's story

> Angela has been trying to make sure her fibroids don't regrow since they were removed six years ago. 'I've been told to try and eat plenty of vegetables to keep my oestrogen levels in check.'

There is increasing interest in phyto-oestrogens, naturally occurring compounds in plants. The key ones, lignans and isoflavones, are similar in structure to oestradiol, the most powerful type of oestrogen produced in the body, but are much weaker. It's claimed that phyto-oestrogens can increase oestrogen-levels when they are too low in the body – for example, in menopausal women: it's been noted that Japanese women, who eat lots of soya beans which are high in plant oestrogens, seem to experience few menopausal symptoms. But it's also claimed that plant oestrogens can lower excessively high oestrogen-levels. If this is the case, then plant oestrogens may help to slow fibroid growth.

Good sources of lignans include linseed, cereal bran, vegetables, peas and beans, vegetables and fruits. The best source of isoflavones is soya and chickpeas.

Summary

- Make sure you get plenty of nuts and seeds, wheatgerm, liver, avocados, peas, beans and leafy greens, potatoes, carrots, seaweed, fruit and fish, as well as soya products.
- Avoid alcohol, which puts more strain on the liver, and sugar and caffeine, which can deplete the body of vital nutrients.
- Also try to cut down saturated fats which come from red meat, eggs and dairy products. A high-fat diet is thought to stress the liver and make it less able to break down oestrogen efficiently, which could contribute to excess oestrogen-levels. You will also lose weight on a low-fat diet, which may keep oestrogen-levels in check.

Pelvic exercises

These are important exercises for women to do throughout life. They are also particularly useful if you have fibroids, because the exercises can improve pelvic circulation and relieve pelvic congestion: fibroids can cause an accumulation of fluid in the pelvis which can be uncomfortable. The exercises also tone up muscles in the pelvis. Several complementary therapists emphasized that it's important to release energy which gets stuck in the pelvis.

Pelvic-floor exercises

The pelvic floor is made up of layers of muscle which support the organs in the pelvis – the bladder, womb and bowel. Women are advised to do these exercises after childbirth, to tone up stretched muscles which may be sagging. These exercises are also worth doing if you have a big, bulky womb with fibroids: they will tone up the pelvic-floor muscles which may be under greater strain. It's also important to get these muscles into good shape in case you have a hysterectomy or myomectomy. Strong, healthy pelvic-floor muscles will also protect against leaky bladders, as well as increasing sexual pleasure.

Learn how to do the pelvic-floor exercises by lying or sitting with your knees slightly apart. Concentrate on the pelvic-floor muscles. Lift and squeeze at the front as if you're trying to stop passing water, and at the back as if you're holding in wind. Hold this contraction for as long as you can – two seconds initially, if possible – and gradually work up to ten seconds. Rest for several seconds, and repeat the sequence about ten times if you can manage it. As you get better at this, try also doing short, fast contractions. Make sure you are exercising the right muscles. Don't hold your breath, or squeeze your buttocks, or tighten your abdominal muscles when doing the exercises. Try and do the exercises a couple of times a day, practising a mixture of slow contractions with pauses and then faster ones. Check that you are using the right muscles by sliding your finger into your vagina when you're doing the exercises. You should feel a gentle squeeze if you're using the right muscles. You can check how strong the muscles are by seeing if you can stop in mid-flow when you are passing urine. Once you have done this, relax and empty your bladder. If your muscles are out of condition, it may take several weeks or months to tone them up.

Pelvic tilt and rock

Pelvic rocking is a good way of improving the circulation in the pelvis. A gentle way to start this is by doing the pelvic tilt. Lie on the floor with your knees bent and feet slightly apart. Pull in your stomach muscles and press the small of your back on to the floor. Hold for a couple of seconds, and then let go; repeat this several times. Check you're doing this properly by putting a hand under the small of your back: you should feel it pressing down on to your hand when you're doing the tilt. You can also practise the pelvic tilt when sitting or standing.

Once you feel confident about doing this, try the pelvic rock. Stand with your feet slightly apart, and then move your pelvis gently from front to back, then from side to side, and finally round in a circle one way and then the other. Experiment, and do what you find most comfortable and enjoyable. As you move, practise contracting the pelvic-floor muscles. Try practising these movements each day for a couple of minutes. However, it's best not to do these exercises if you are having your period because they may increase blood-flow.

Deep breathing for the pelvis

One complementary therapist I spoke to said that deep abdominal breathing could help improve circulation in the pelvis. Lie on the floor with a cushion under your buttocks, with your knees bent and feet together. Open your knees and let them drop gently to either side of your body as far as they will comfortably go. You'll end up with the soles of your feet facing each other. Put your hands on your lower abdomen and think of breathing into that area for several minutes.

Also, try sitting upright on the floor with your knees bent, feet together. Again, let your knees drop gently to either side as far as they will comfortably go. Place a hand on each knee and stay in this position for a few minutes while doing some deep abdominal breathing. Make sure you are not breathing high up in your chest. If you're doing anything strenuous, you use the upper part of your lungs – but normally, you should breathe lower down. This helps relaxation and is good for health. (This is discussed in more detail later in the chapter, in the section on stress.)

Weight control

If you're very overweight, your body may be producing more oestrogen, which could be contributing to your fibroid problems. Even if this theory proves to be incorrect, it still makes sense to slim down: if you're very overweight, surgery may be more risky and recovery time could be longer. Lose weight by eating a healthy, low-fat diet, as discussed earlier on, and by taking plenty of exercise.

119

Exercise

Exercise is important because it improves circulation generally, and increases your sense of well-being. People who exercise regularly experience less tension, fatigue, and depression, and are better able to deal with stress. If you are fit, you will recover more quickly from surgery. Physical activity also protects against heart disease and strokes.

But many of us lead sedentary lives and don't exercise. If you find the idea of getting fit or of sport offputting, think about being active and doing something you enjoy: walking, gardening, cycling, dancing and swimming are all good ways of getting moving.

Stress

A certain amount of stress is good for us, as it helps us avoid danger and lead life to the full. Our bodies react in a certain way – known as the fight-flight response – when we face threats or challenges. Various stress-hormones are released, which help us get going in the morning and achieve our goals.

But chronic, long-term stress isn't helpful, and is linked to a range of health problems – such as high blood-pressure and stomach problems. Prolonged stress can make you feel unwell – and it also seems to affect hormonal balance. There is plenty of anecdotal evidence that stressful events, such as bereavement, can affect periods in all sorts of ways. Periods may stop altogether, or may become much heavier. You may also experience more pain.

Sarah's story

Sarah thinks that stress contributed to her increased bleeding, and wonders whether this was responsible for her period problems, rather than her fibroids. 'The very heavy bleeding coincided with a difficult time at the office last year, when I was very busy and also having problems with one of my colleagues.'

Some researchers also claim that stress is linked to eggless cycles which are characterized by oestrogen dominance.

Warning signs of being over-stressed include tense muscles, diarrhoea, constipation, migraines, skin problems, tiredness and sleep problems. You may find yourself having mood swings, bursting into tears and feeling depressed, anxious and fearful. You may want to smoke and drink more and find it difficult to concentrate and finish tasks.

There are various benefits to be gained from being less stressed. You will feel more cheerful and positive, and be more able to cope with fibroid symptoms, which in turn may seem less severe. Recovery from surgery is also likely to be quicker if you are less stressed. Stress-levels can be reduced through practising relaxation techniques, such as yoga, meditation and visualization. It's a question of experimenting and finding out what suits you. Alongside this you also need to take sufficient rest and exercise, and have a healthy diet.

Tips for managing stress

The starting point is to recognize that you are under a lot of stress, and that you perhaps need to make some changes in your life. Negative thinking can also become a habit. Laughter also helps because it reduces muscle tension, regulates the heartbeat and improves breathing.

Change what you can change, and try to accept those things that you cannot change. Try not to let everything pile up, and deal with one thing at a time. If possible, try to avoid a lot of major changes all at once. Talk about how you feel, and don't bottle things up: you may find it useful to see a counsellor. Try to be realistic about what you can achieve.

Correct breathing

Learning to breathe correctly can help to reduce stress. Prolonged stress can make people hyperventilate – which means overbreathing. Rapid, shallow breathing using the upper chest muscles is normal during strenuous exercise, but it is unnecessary to use these muscles for ordinary activity. Your carbon dioxide levels will drop too low if you routinely use your upper chest to breathe. This can change the normal alkaline/acid balance in the blood. You may experience various symptoms, such as chest pain, panicky feelings, anxiety and bowel disturbance.

Use the diaphragm – the sheet of muscle which separates the chest from the abdomen – for normal, everyday breathing. Check how you are breathing by lying on the floor, and putting one hand on the waist area and the other on the upper chest. When you breathe in, you should notice the hand on your waist moving upwards rather than the hand on your upper chest.

Relaxation techniques

There are various ways of unwinding. Lie down in a quiet, warm room where you won't be disturbed for 20 minutes or so. Working from your feet upwards through your body, check for signs of muscle-tension and let go of it. Repeat to yourself: 'I feel heavy and warm'. If thoughts crowd into your mind, note them – but just accept the thoughts passing through.

Meditation can help relax the mind and body. It's a calming technique in which you focus on one object or word. Again, allow yourself about 20 minutes to do this. Concentrate on a word or image which you have chosen, and keep going back to it if other thoughts intrude.

Massage on a regular basis can also help you relax and forget your worries. Digestion is better, blood-pressure is lower and breathing slows down after a good massage.

Yoga is well worth considering, as it can help calm both mind and body, as well as toning up muscles. Yoga exercises which focus on the pelvis can also help reduce pelvic congestion and low back-pain. The slow, controlled stretching movements can help to relax tense muscles and promote suppleness, so improving blood circulation and oxygenation in the pelvis. Yoga therapy focuses on exercises which can help stress-related conditions, and also period problems and menopausal symptoms.

Visualization exercises can help stimulate positive chemical and hormonal changes, according to some researchers. They think that the power of the mind can heal disease. In an American magazine article written in the late 1980s, a woman described how she had used these techniques to get rid of her fibroid. For several months she went through a daily session of deep relaxation. She became aware of her breathing and let tension flow out of her body. When she was deeply relaxed, she imagined sharks eating her fibroid. She returned to see her gynaecologist for a check-up some months later. The fibroid had disappeared – so there was no need for the hysterectomy which she had originally been advised was necessary.

122

The contraceptive Pill

The usefulness of the Pill as a treatment for heavy bleeding was discussed in Chapter 6 – we saw there that it may not be so effective when these problems are caused by fibroids. But apart from the issue of whether the Pill is helpful as a medical treatment, there is no reason why you should not take the Pill as your preferred method of contraception. Other factors – such as your health and age – will determine whether you can take the Pill, and which one is best for you.

HRT

If you're coming up to the menopause and have troublesome fibroids, then HRT may be of particular concern to you. This was certainly so for several of the women I spoke to. In Chapter 5, we considered the differing opinions as to whether you should take HRT if you've had troublesome fibroids. Some gynaecologists argue that it can be safely prescribed, provided the fibroids are properly monitored. A few doctors may not be willing to prescribe HRT unless you have a hysterectomy – and if this is the case, you could always consider consulting another doctor for a second opinion.

Alternatives to HRT

HRT is currently very popular. Many doctors argue that it is the best way to treat distressing menopausal symptoms, such as hot flushes and vaginal dryness – and the only way effectively to protect against bone-thinning problems and heart disease in later life. HRT is being promoted as a supplement which women should automatically take when their hormone-levels change, regardless of whether or not they are actually experiencing significant menopausal problems.

But some doctors worry that HRT can cause side-effects, such as mood changes, and also that women may become addicted to HRT – though it's claimed that these problems can be sorted out by trying out a different type of HRT. These doctors also want to know about the possible harmful side-effects of taking HRT long-term.

What should you do if you don't want to take HRT because you have symptom-causing fibroids, but are worried about the prospect of menopausal symptoms? It's best to talk through your concerns with your doctor. Some women experience few menopausal problems: if you are in this group you may see no need to take HRT – though there are still longer-term health issues to consider, notably heart disease and osteoporosis. HRT is currently promoted as being vital for women's health after the menopause. But some complementary therapists think that there are other ways of treating menopausal symptoms. They argue that some types of oestrogen go on being produced in the body after the menopause, and that various measures can be used to help women through the menopause as well as protecting against long-term problems. Contrary to conventional wisdom, a few people also argue that menopausal problems are caused by a lack of progesterone rather than oestrogen. They therefore advocate taking natural progesterone supplements. However, this theory also needs critical examination as these supplements may have side-effects.

An alternative approach to HRT consists of advice about a healthy diet, as outlined earlier, as well as keeping stress under control and practising relaxation techniques.

Specific advice would be to eat plenty of plant oestrogens, such as soya and linseed, to help the body make the hormonal adjustments experienced at the menopause and to minimize side-effects. Herbs such as *vitex agnus castus*, *dong quai* and wild yam are often used to help this adjustment. You can buy these yourself, but it's much better to see a herbalist for most effective help.

Hot flushes can be minimized by making sure you get plenty of vitamin E in your diet. Wear clothes you can easily adjust if you have a hot flush. Also, try to avoid stimulants such as coffee and tea, and set time aside each day to practise relaxation techniques. A diet rich in vitamin B can help mood swings. Vitamin E, orgasm, love-making, and pelvic exercises can all help vaginal dryness. Research also shows that vitamin E can help protect against heart disease. Menopausal supplements are available from chemists – but it's best to consult a nutritional therapist for advice.

You also need to make sure you keep your bones strong to reduce the risk of developing osteoporosis. You can do this by giving up smoking and taking plenty of weight-bearing exercise several times a week (such as walking, skipping or dancing). You should also eat lots of calcium-rich foods and keep alcohol intake down, as alcohol prevents calcium from being absorbed into the body. The daily recommended calcium intake is 1,500 mg if you are over 45. Good sources of calcium include low-fat dairy products, canned fish, nuts and dark green vegetables.

You can also have a bone-scan if you think you are at special risk of developing osteoporosis and need medical treatment – for example, if you have suffered a fracture after a minor bump or fall, as strong bones wouldn't normally break; if there is a family history of the disease; if you have taken steroid drugs for a long time or you have suffered from conditions such as thyroid disease.

Summary

- Make sure that you are not anaemic, and if you are, get treatment.
- Have a healthy diet.
- Do pelvic exercises.
- Lose excess weight.
- Keep stress under control.
- The contraceptive Pill can be taken if you have fibroids (though of course there may be other reasons why you can't take the Pill).
- HRT can usually be taken, but if you don't want to take it, there are other ways of dealing with menopausal symptoms.

Useful addresses

Acupuncture

Acupuncture Council
Park House
206 Latimer Road
London W10 6RE
0181 964 0222

Contraceptive Pill queries

Family Planning Association
2–12 Pentonville Road
London N1 9FP
0171 837 4044

Herbalism

The National Institute of Medical Herbalists
56 Longbrook Street
Exeter EX4 6AH
01392 426022

Homeopathy

British Homoeopathic Association
27a Devonshire Street
London WlN lRJ
0171 935 2163

Hormone replacement therapy queries

The Amarant Trust
11–13 Charterhouse Buildings
London EClM 7AN
0171 490 1644

Infertility support and information groups

CHILD
Charter House
43 St Leonards Road
Bexhill on Sea
East Sussex TN40 1JA
01424 732361

ISSUE

The National Fertility Association
509 Aldridge Road
Great Barr
Birmingham B44 8NA
0121 344 4414

Nutrition

If you want to see a dietician, ask your GP if you can be referred to one.
For a nutritional therapist contact:
Society for the Promotion of Nutritional Therapy
P O Box 47
Heathfield
East Sussex TN21 8ZX
01435 867007

Physiotherapy

Chartered Society of Physiotherapy
14 Bedford Row
London WClR 4ED
0171 242 1941

Queries on patient's rights

Association of Community Health Councils
30 Drayton Park
London N5 1PB
0171 609 8405

Queries – general

Healthpoint NHS information line
Freephone 0800 665544

Royal College of Obstetricians and Gynaecologists Bookshop

78 Park Road
London NW1
0171 772 6275

The Wel (Women's Endoscopic Laser) Foundation

South Cleveland Hospital
Marton Road
Middlesbrough
Cleveland TS4 3BW
01642 820070

Women's Health run telephone inquiry line
0171 251 6580

Yoga

Yoga Therapy Centre
Royal London Homoeopathic Hospital
Great Ormond Street
London 0171 833 7267

Further reading

Brewer, Sarah, *Endometriosis and Fibroids*. Vermilion, 1995.

Butterworth, Jane, *Hysterectomy*. Thorsons, 1995.

Davies, Jill, *Anaemia*. Thorsons, 1993.

Grant, Rosalind, *Which? Medicine*, Which? Books, 1995.

Lark, Susan, *Fibroid Tumors & Endometriosis*. Celestial Arts, 1995.

MacGregor, Anne, *Is HRT Right for You?* Sheldon Press, 1993.

Melville, Arabella, *Natural Hormone Health*. Thorsons, 1990.

Nissim, Rina, *Natural Healing in Gynaecology*. Pandora Press, 1986.

Shaw, R. S., *Uterine Fibroids, Time for Review*. Parthenon Publishing Group, 1992.

Smart, Felicity, with Professor Stuart Campbell, *Fibroids: the Latest Treatment Options for this Common Problem*. Thorsons, 1993.

Woodham, Anne, *HEA Guide to Complementary Medicine and Therapies*. Health Education Authority, 1994.

Vassallo, Catherine, *The Good Doctor Guide*. Simon & Schuster, 1997.

Index